Testimonials

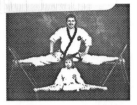

"Thanks for your Secrets of Stretching VHS cassette. At first I wasn't sure it could happen to me, but nothing can be totally impossible!"—Dave Walk

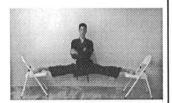

"After using your method for 3 months everyday, I have achieved the side split in suspension. In addition, my kicking techniques have become higher and much stronger."—Elias P. Bonaros, Jr.

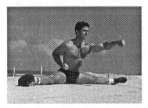

"Enclosed you will find two photos with results achieved with your method"—Yoel Ben-Aroch

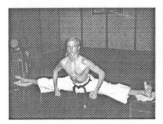

"I can't believe how well your book works! I have never been able to achieve the full splits or have as much strength as your method has given me. Here is my picture, just so you'll know how well it worked for me. This doesn't even hurt!"—Matt Summers

"...we instituted your exercises within our class structure and not surprisingly, almost all of our students increased flexibility in a few months. The ad said 'It could be your picture...' Well, enclosed is actual photo with proof positive that your method does produce results."—Stephen Dileo

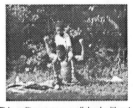

"This split was accomplished without a warm-up. I attribute that capability to your method. It not only has increased the height of my kicks and flexibility in the legs but also strength in lifting. I can squat heavier, more reps, and recover faster with your stretching method."—Ken Nero

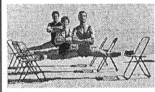

"Don't talk... Stop laughing guys... People will think you laugh at other experts.... It is not nice... Get serious, okay... I haven't got a whole day! Don't move! Okay."—Photographer

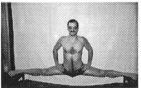

"I am pleased with this system, why wasn't the book written 15 years ago!"—George Patnoe, Jr.

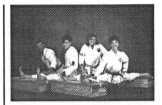

"The results have been astounding! Students have displayed excellent flexibility which they parlayed into outstanding kicks in terms of height, speed, and power. Additional benefits have occurred. For instance... injury rates have declined significantly."—Stephen Dileo

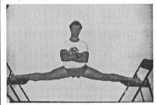

"I have had your stretching book for a couple of years and was able to do the side splits after a couple of months. I was satisfied with that accomplishment until the beginning of this past summer. I decided to do the "impossible," the split between the chairs. Enclosed is my photo. I totally agree with your statement, in the magazines, "An 'authority' that can't show this [the split between chairs] is no authority." Thanks, your method does work, & it's the best"—Mike Adrowski

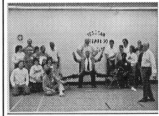

Without any warm-up Tom Kurz performs a side split on chairs while explaining benefits of his method of stretching to martial arts instructors, in Essex Junction, VT at the meeting of Vermont Martial Arts Association in June 1992.

Stretching Scientifically

A Guide to Flexibility Training

by Thomas Kurz, M. Sc.

Third edition, completely revised

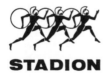

STADION

Stretching Scientifically
A Guide to Flexibility Training

by Thomas Kurz, M.Sc.

Published by:

STADION

Stadion Publishing Company, Inc.
Post Office Box 447
Island Pond, VT 05846, U.S.A.

Publisher's Cataloging in Publication
(Prepared by Quality Books Inc.)

Kurz, Thomas, 1956-
Stretching scientifically: a guide to flexibility training /
Thomas Kurz. — [New ed.]
p. cm.
Bibliography: p. 137
Includes index
ISBN 0-940149-30-3 (paper trade)
ISBN 0-940149-29-X (library binding)

1. Physical education and training. 2. Physical fitness. 3. Stretching exercises. I. Title
GV711.5.K87 1987   613.7'1
                                        92-85420

Editing by R. Scott Perry
Cover and Book Design by Eva Chodkiewicz-Swider
Photography by Chuck Shahood

I dedicate this book to Antoni Zagorski and Tadeusz Sadowski. Without their help it would have never been written.

About the author

Before coming to the U.S.A., Thomas Kurz studied physical education in one of the top East European institutions that prepare coaches, instructors, teachers of physical education, and rehabilitation specialists.

He studied for five years at Akademia Wychowania Fizycznego (Academy of Physical Education) in Warsaw. While still a student, he was appointed assistant coach of the students' judo team. A versatile athlete, Kurz competed in several Olympic sports, including swimming, gymnastics, and track and field events. This versatility shows itself now in his expertise in the field of sports methodology and physical education, an expertise evident in his work with his students, as well as in this book.

Mark Bazylko, M.Sc.
Judo Coach, Former National Team Member (Poland)

Acknowledgments

Everything I know about physical education, sports, and training, I have learned from teachers at Akademia Wychowania Fizycznego (Academy of Physical Education). They taught me the most modern (if something so advanced can be called merely modern) methods of training. To them, and all East Bloc P.E. teachers and coaches, this book is nothing new, because all I did was put in writing what they have been teaching for many years. I am especially grateful to my teachers for bringing the importance of methodology in physical education and sports to the attention of me and my fellow students.

Preface

In this book you will find all the information about flexibility training that you need to succeed in sports.

My first book on this subject, published in 1985, was a great success. Several readers wrote me about the gains they had made thanks to my instruction. There were readers, though, who either had difficulty understanding these instructions, fitting the exercises into their training, or who after initial rapid gains reached a level well short of their goal (and their potential) and could not progress any further. Using the feedback from all these readers, I completely rewrote the book. It is now even more understandable and more informative.

If you have read only the books and research papers on flexibility that were published in the West, you will notice that I sometimes use different terms in writing about this subject. Other times familiar terms may denote something different than the meaning you are used to. This is so because I was trained in a completely different system of physical education and sports. The terms I use are a direct translation of the terms used in the East bloc's physical education and sports methodology.

With the collapse of the Soviet Union, the term *East bloc* is rapidly assuming a status of quaint antiquity. It was used to refer to the nations of Eastern Europe that had been unwillingly absorbed by the U.S.S.R. For decades these nations—especially Poland, East Germany, Hungary, and Rumania—dominated Olympic and other international athletic contests far beyond what one might expect based on size and resources. The difference lay in their common use of advanced methods of training.

The Methodology of P.E. and Sports is the central subject in university courses for coaches and P.E. teachers there. The knowledge of it makes all the difference between success and failure in developing athletic skills and abilities, or simply, getting results from one's exercises. In describing the methods of stretching, I have given as much information about the correct ways of working out as possible without making this book a complete manual on the methodology of physical education.

TABLE OF CONTENTS

1. Theory

You most likely already know what flexibility is and what the advantages are to having it developed to a high level. It is one of the essential motor qualities of an athlete. A high level of flexibility helps one to perform more economically in fencing, judo, wrestling, and other sports. Certain sports—e.g., gymnastics, javelin throw, kickboxing—require a maximal development of it just for the execution of their basic techniques.

Some motor qualities are inborn, such as speed; others, such as balance, have to be developed at a certain age to reach an exceptional level. Flexibility is like strength and endurance, however, in that it can be brought to high levels by anybody and at any time in one's life. Outside of pathological cases, there is no such thing as inborn flexibility.

You can improve flexibility by doing exercises such as running, swimming, and weightlifting as long as your limbs go through the full range of motion. Not all athletes can always lift weights or run middle and long distances, though. At some stages of training, these exercises can interfere with the development of their special form. Properly chosen stretching exercises are less time- and energy-consuming than these indirect methods.

Apart from increasing the range of movement in your joints, stretching has other functions in your workout. At the beginning of the workout, some dynamic stretches can be good warm-up exercises. At the end of it, stretching facilitates recovery: regulating muscular tension, relieving muscle spasms, and improving blood flow in muscles. It also makes a great cool-down exercise.

In this chapter, you will learn most of the whys of stretching. This method of developing flexibility works regardless of whether or not you understand its physiological basis, as long as you do the exercises exactly as prescribed in chapters 2-6. Nevertheless, the more you know, the better your choice of exercises and the likelihood of getting the results you want. Information—good information!—also gives you the basis for countering bad advice you may receive. Note this well: Mental rigidity—the inability to abandon fixed ideas—is usually accompanied by a low level of physical flexibility.

A description of the body organs that dictate how flexible you are is a good place to start.

Skeletal muscle consists of many muscle fibers (cells) arranged in parallel bundles. Muscles can grow in diameter by increasing the thickness and number of miofibrils, and in length by forming additional sarcomeres—the functional units of a muscle cell. They have the ability to contract, and if relaxed, are very extensible. When a muscle contracts, two kinds of protein (actin and myosin) in the sarcomeres of its cells slide along one another. In the body, a muscle can be contracted to 70% or stretched to 130% of its normal resting length. (Normal resting length is the length that the muscle takes up in the body in a typical resting attitude.) Outside the body, the muscle can be contracted to 50% of its length and stretched more than 130%. As a muscle is stretched beyond its normal resting length, its force of contraction gradually drops, reaching zero at 175% of resting length. The diminishing strength of contraction is caused by a decreasing amount of overlap between actin and myosin.

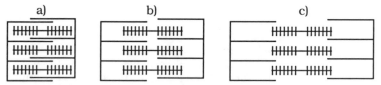

Amount of overlap of actin and myosin in a sarcomere
a) of contracted, b) resting, and c) stretched muscle

Muscle contracts with greatest force at its normal resting length. Whole muscle is encased in a fibrous connective tissue sheath (epimysium). Bundles and even single cells are also surrounded by the same tissue (perimysium and endomysium). The tension generated by muscle cells is transferred to the fibers of connective tissue.

Tendons are cordlike extensions of this tissue. Collagen fibers, a major element of fibrous connective tissue, have great strength, little extensibility, and no ability to contract. These fibers are arranged in wavy bundles allowing motion until the slack of these bundles is taken up. Extension of a tendon beyond four percent of its length causes irreversible deformation. An improper use of isometric or eccentric tensions can put too much stress on collagen fibers, damaging them and causing muscle soreness—a result of the disintegration of collagen and the release of hydroxyproline (one of its components) into the muscle. With age, molecules of collagen change by becoming more rigid, which is reflected in general body stiffness.

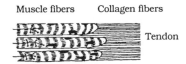

Collagen fibers surrounding muscle fibers at their junction with the tendon

You can permanently elongate tendons and connective tissue sheaths, with minimal structural weakening by low-force long-duration stretching with temperatures of the tendons at more than 103°F. To increase the amount of permanent elongation, you maintain the stretch achieved while tendons and sheaths were warm while they cool down. This fits the description of a relaxed stretch done after the main part of your workout during the cool-down, with this qualifier: the stretch must be at the range of motion at which muscle fibers exert less tension than the connective tissue.

The joint capsule is a connective tissue sleeve that completely surrounds each movable joint. Immobilization for a few weeks causes chemical changes in the collagen fibers of the joint capsule that will restrict your flexibility.

The ligaments holding your joints together are made primarily of collagen fibers. They have more elastic fibers, made of the protein elastin, than do tendons. Stretching ligaments leads to loose-jointedness and can be effectively applied only with children. In adults, an age-related increase in rigidity of collagen fibers makes any stretches aimed at elongating ligaments hazardous. When children stretch ballistically or statically, their muscles do not contract as strongly as an adult's and their ligaments can be stretched. If a ligament is stretched more than six percent of its normal length, it tears. There is no need to stretch ligaments to perform even the most spectacular karate or gymnastic techniques. The natural range of motion is sufficient. Stretching ligaments destabilizes joints and thus may cause osteoarthritis (Beighton, Grahame, and Bird 1983).

Bone is a dynamic, living tissue made of crystals of calcium and phosphorus that are associated with collagen fibers. Exercises can change the density and shape of bones. The forms of joint surfaces, covered by a glasslike, smooth and elastic cartilage, also change in the long-term process of exercise, e.g., dynamic stretching. Depending on the amount of stress (exercise, for example), bones and joints can adapt to it or be destroyed by it.

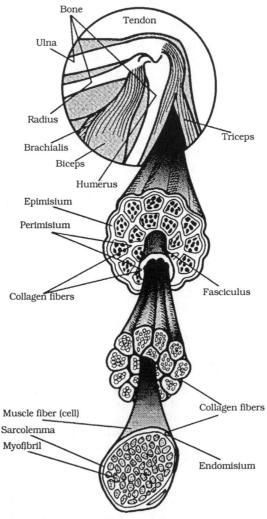

Cross-section through a skeletal muscle

Here are simple tests to convince you that the structure of joints and the length of ligaments does not keep you from doing splits.

Front split. If the angle between the front and rear leg is less than 180 degrees with the front leg straight, flex the knee of your front leg and see what happens.

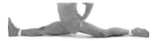

Front split with front leg straight

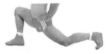

Deep lunge. The knee of the front leg is flexed and the angle between thighs is 180 degrees.

If you started to stretch past the age when elongating ligaments was possible, you probably have difficulty touching the ground with the front thigh of the rear leg in this split. What keeps you from doing this is usually not a muscle, but a ligament (lig. iliofemorale) running in front of your hip joint. It is tightened by an extension of the hip (posterior tilting of the pelvis or moving the thigh to the back while keeping the pelvis straight). Flexing the hip (tilting the pelvis forward or moving the thigh to the front) relaxes this ligament. To achieve a nice, flat split you need to stretch the hamstring of the front leg and the muscles of the lower back so you can tilt the pelvis forward while keeping the trunk upright. To make sure that the muscles (hip flexors) pulling your thigh forward are not exceptionally short, do this test: Lie on a table, on your back, with your lower legs hanging over the edge. Pull one leg, with its knee flexed, toward your chest. Keep your back flat on the table. If the other leg, left lying on the table, is lifted by this movement before the angle between your thighs reaches 120 degrees, your iliopsoas (hip flexor) needs some stretching.

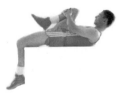

Iliopsoas length test

Side split. A person unable to do a complete split can bring one of the thighs into the position it would have in relation to the hip in the split, or at least get it much closer to this position than when spreading both legs at the same time. No muscles run from one leg to another. If you can do one half of the split, only the reflexive contraction of the muscles (and not the ligaments, or the muscles' connective tissue sheaths) prevents you from doing a complete split with equal ease.

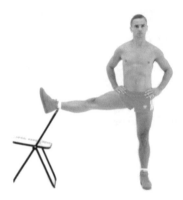

If you think that the structure of your hips will not let you do side splits, try this test. The leg resting on the chair is in the position it would have in a split.

Note that in doing a side split you not only spread the legs sideways, but also you tilt the pelvis forward (push buttocks to the rear). In a side split with the feet pointing up, you keep your pelvis straight but rotate the thighs outward. The alignment of the hips and thighs in both types of the side split is the same. You cannot do this split without either rotating your thighs outward or tilting the pelvis forward. This forward tilt (hip flexion) unwinds capsular ligaments of the hip, among them the pubofemoral ligament, which resist excessive abduction. Spreading the legs without these additional movements twists and tightens the ligaments of the hip and jams the necks of the thigh bones against the brim of the joint cavity of your pelvis. (A similar ease-of-movement technique happens in the shoulder joint—you can move your arm further back or up if you rotate your arm because this allows the greater tuberosity of the humerus to pass behind the acromion, a bony process on top of the shoulder blade, instead of hitting it.)

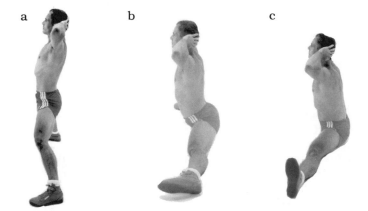

a) Starting position for a side split
b) Getting into a side split: legs are spread sideways and hips tilt to the rear
c) Side split with feet pointing up. The hips are straight thanks to rotation of the thighs.

The amount of outside rotation of the femur in the hip decides the quality of your side split. It is limited by the gluteus medius, gluteus minimus, psoas major, and the posterior belly of adductor magnus, all muscles that rotate the thigh inside. Normally adductors pull the thigh inward and rotate it outward, but if the thigh is rotated outward as much as it takes to do a side split or a first ballet position, adductors also help to rotate it inward. It means that in addition to being stretched by abduction they are also stretched by the extreme outside rotation and can limit this rotation.

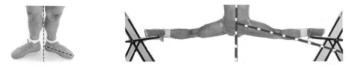

Outside rotation of the thigh in first ballet position. Nearly 90 degrees of turnout of the foot are achieved by 60 to 70 degrees of external rotation at the hip, with the remaining 20 to 30 degrees accounted for by the natural outward inclination of the knee and the foot-ankle complex. Note the relation of the angle (less than 90 degrees from the centerline) in this position, to the angle (less than 180 degrees) between the thighs in a side split.

In the preceding examples, relieving the tension of the muscles around the joint increases its range of motion. This means that only muscular tension prevents you from doing splits. Muscular tension has two components: the tension generated by the contractile elements (muscle fibers); and the tension present even in an inactive, denervated muscle, exerted by the connective tissues associated with the muscle. Some authors (M. J. Alter, B. Anderson, H. A. deVries, S. A. Sölveborn) declare the connective tissue tension to be the main factor restricting flexibility. They advocate slow static stretching, even in a warm-up, as if muscles were pieces of fabric to be elongated to a desired size. Robert W. Ramsey and Sibil F. Street (1940) prove and state it clearly that if the range of extension does not exceed the 130% of resting length, the resting tension in a noncontracting muscle is very small. (You remember that 130% of resting length is usually the maximum stretch of a muscle in the body.) Shottelius and Senay (1956) show that in the muscle stretched to well over 100% of its resting length the passive tension generated by its connective tissue is a small fraction of the tension due to active contraction. They show that eventually, at approximately 120% of a muscle's resting length, the two components of muscle tension contribute equally to total tension. At greater lengths the passive tension increases while the active tension, generated by contracting muscle fibers, decreases. For practical purposes, as long as you feel your muscles contract in response to a stretch, it means that relaxing the contractile elements can improve your stretch and that you should concern yourself more with nervous regulation of your muscles' tension and less with your muscles' connective tissue. The side split test shown on page 16 proves it neatly.

The nervous system regulates tension and thus the relative length of your muscles by influencing the contractile element. (The illustration on page 21 sums up what follows.) Several nerve cells receive signals from and send signals to each muscle. Nerve cells receiving the signals are called *afferent* or sensory neurons. Directly, or through other neurons, they contact nerve cells that send signals to the muscles. The cells whose axons (nerve fibers) conduct signals to the muscles are called *efferent* or motoneurons. Their cell bodies are located in the spinal cord or in the brainstem. Other neurons contact and influence motoneurons. Some can stimulate the motoneurons, which causes a contraction of the muscle fibers innervated by them. Some can inhibit (block) motoneurons, causing a relaxation of muscle fibers. When the motoneurons of one set of muscles are stimulated, motoneurons of the muscles opposing them are inhibited. This is called *reciprocal inhibition*. It allows you to move. Neurons causing contraction of muscles are called motoneurons Alpha. Doing dynamic stretches as a warm-up for a dynamic action requires stimulating motoneurons of the moving, contracting muscles in a way that is similar to the stimulation they will receive during the action. During static stretches those motoneurons are not stimulated in such a way.

Muscle spindles are embedded within a muscle. They consist of special kinds of muscle fibers that can contract only at their ends. At their center are the stretch receptors. There are two kinds of stretch receptors: one, characterized by flower-spray and spiral endings mainly on nuclear chain fibers, responding only to the magnitude of the stretch; another, with annulospiral endings on both nuclear bag and chain fibers, that responds to both the magnitude and the speed of stretching. Muscle spindles in a stretched muscle send signals that reach a motoneuron Alpha and cause it to send impulses to the muscle. For example, when a muscle is stretched by tapping its tendon as in testing the knee-jerk reflex, receptors in the spindles send impulses that reach motoneurons Alpha, stimulating the contraction of this muscle and its *synergists*, or cooperating muscles. The same impulse, sent by stretch receptors, inhibits muscles antagonistic to it, and so your leg kicks. This knee-jerk reflex is an example of a myotatic or stretch reflex. Every stretch causes a contraction preventing further stretching. This contraction lowers the stimulation of the spindles. Isometric contraction decreases the frequency of signals from muscle spindle (Bishop 1982).

There are neural circuits and pathways that can cause lessened resistance to stretch, more formally called *postcontractive reflex depression*. Postcontractive reflex depression follows a strong voluntary contraction of the muscle about to be stretched. It permits a greater range of motion increase than stretching without a preceding contraction. No matter what the exact cause of lessening the resistance to stretch, the resistance is smallest within the first second of relaxation after a contraction and then recovers to nearly 70% of its normal values by the fifth second (Moore and Kukulka 1991). This means that your stretch is easiest within the first second after the end of a contraction.

Motoneurons Gamma are located in the spinal cord, close to motoneurons Alpha. These neurons regulate the tension of muscle spindles, so that if the whole muscle is contracted, the spindle can adjust and still be able to detect changes in muscle length.

The brain, through its pathways of nerve fibers conducting impulses downwards, similarly affects motoneurons Alpha and Gamma, but the Gamma are more sensitive. Gamma motoneurons, which regulate the muscle spindles' detection of the magnitude of a stretch, are stimulated by the cold center and inhibited by the heat center in your hypothalamus. Motoneurons Gamma are thus easier to activate when your body temperature is low and so your flexibility worsens then. Pain, anxiety, and fear, thanks to these same descending pathways, also activate motoneurons Gamma, thus making you less flexible (Sölveborn 1989). This is one more reason not to do static passive stretches during a warm-up when you may be excited or even anxious about the challenging activities ahead.

Descending pathways, motoneurons Gamma, spindle muscle fibers, stretch receptors (in a particular spindle), sensory neurons (innervating a particular spindle), and motoneuron Alpha are collectively called the Gamma loop. The Gamma loop activity measures and influences the length and tension of a muscle. Thanks to this loop, the same weight can be supported by different lengths of a muscle or, the same length can support different weights. The Gamma loop regulates the sensitivity of muscle spindles. If, because of lowered tonus, an insufficient amount of impulses comes from stretch receptors, the Gamma loop compensates, making the muscle spindles shorter. That is why people experience stiffness upon first awakening.

Apart from the Gamma loop, muscular tension is regulated by the Golgi organs and the Renshaw cells.

The Golgi organs are located in the tendon at its junction with the muscle. The contracting muscle pulls on the tendon causing the Golgi organs to fire impulses in relation to the force of contraction. These impulses activate association neurons, which then send their impulses to inhibit the motoneurons Alpha of the contracting muscle. This stops the flow of impulses from motoneuron Alpha to the muscle. (This is the usual explanation for the mechanism of PNF [Proprioceptive Neuromuscular Facilitation] and isometric stretching.) Some Golgi organs have high thresholds and act as a safety feature in case of excessive contraction or excessive stretching. The rest of the Golgi organs, having a lower threshold, supply the motor centers with information about the tension of the muscle. The Golgi organs that have a high threshold are the ones causing the greatest relaxation. The Golgi organs may also influence motoneurons Gamma.

Renshaw cells are small nerve cells located close to the motoneurons Alpha. They are connected through synapses with motoneurons and are activated by the impulses that these motoneurons send to muscle fibers. Renshaw cells through their axons synapse back both on the motoneurons that activate them and on others. Impulses from the Renshaw cells inhibit motoneurons. This circuit regulates the frequency of impulses received by muscles and keeps them from making contractions that are too strong. Renshaw cells are connected with both the small (tonic) motoneurons Alpha innervating slow-twitch muscle fibers and with the large (phasic) motoneurons Alpha innervating fast-twitch muscle fibers. Renshaw cells are more strongly excited by impulses from phasic motoneurons activated in voluntary contractions than by impulses from tonic motoneurons, but when excited they inhibit tonic motoneurons, most responsive to myotatic or stretch reflex, much more than phasic ones. This is another possible explanation of isometric stretching.

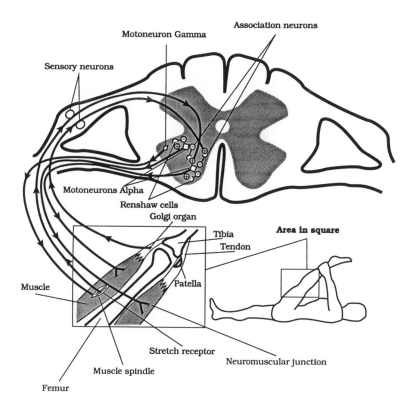

Structures and nerve pathways involved in control of a muscle at the level of its corresponding segment of spinal cord

Your kinesthetic, or muscle, sense is served by more than the already described kinds of receptors (muscle spindles and Golgi organs).

- Pacinian corpuscles, rapidly adapting receptors, are found in the skin and sheaths of muscles and in tendons close to Golgi organs. In the skin they detect vibrations; in other organs they also detect deep pressure and quick movement.
- Ruffini endings, slowly adapting receptors, sense pressure.
- Three kinds of receptors are located in the capsules of your joints.
— Free nerve endings sense joint pain
— Ruffini endings, slowly adapting receptors, are scattered throughout the joint capsule, and sense the position of the joint.
— Paciniform endings, rapidly adapting receptors, sense the direction and speed of motion.

The combined input from all the receptors influences reflexive reactions to the changes in your body position and muscular tension. Your actual reflexes are never as simple as the oversimplified description of a knee-jerk. Usually the whole body responds to any stimulus. Remember the test (see page 16) where you could see if the bones and ligaments of your hips would let you do a side split? There is no muscle or ligament running from one thigh to another, yet, without some training, you cannot do a complete side split! When you spread both legs at the same time, the reflexive contraction of the muscles, on both sides of the body, gets in your way. Reflexes serve useful purposes in normal circumstances and, when your legs slide sideways, the tension of the adductors and their synergists on both sides of the body is needed to maintain posture.

So much for the reflexive regulation of muscular tension. Now consider the brain's role in control of muscular tension through either stimulating or inhibiting motoneurons.

The Proprioceptive-Cerebellar System: Some of the nerve fibers conducting kinesthetic information go to the cerebellum where, without your being aware of it, your tonus, coordination, and balance are regulated. Other fibers go to the cerebral cortex, the outer layer of the brain, which contains higher centers that interpret and correlate sensory data. These fibers provide you with sensory data you are conscious of: the data you feel. The neurons located in the cerebral cortex contact motoneurons through the descending pathways.

The direct descending pathway (pyramidal tract) consists of nerve fibers originating in the cerebral cortex and ending in the spinal cord. These fibers synapse on the motoneurons Alpha, Gamma, and association neurons. This direct pathway governs precise, voluntary movements. Through conscious decisions to make certain movements or to contract groups of muscles, you can override some of your reflexes.

In the multineuronal descending pathway (extrapyramidal tract), neurons from the cerebral cortex synapse through their axons with neurons in the subcortical centers (nerve centers below the cortex) and in the cerebellum. The latter eventually synapse either on association neurons or on motoneurons Gamma. This pathway is responsible for the control of rapid movements, postural mechanisms, the coordination of simultaneous movements of locomotion, and the coordination of fine voluntary movements with postural mechanisms. The connection between the cerebellum and the areas of the brain governing emotions (hippocampus, amygdala, septal areas), makes muscular tonus and coordination dependent on emotions, and vice versa.

Yoga uses this connection. Yoga exercises (asanas) do not use tension in a stretched position. By holding relaxed muscles in a position just short of pain and reflexive contraction, Yogis (in a long-term process) gradually lower the sensitivity of the mechanisms regulating the tension and length of the muscles. Yoga stretches seem to be a litmus test, or a sort of biofeedback monitor, telling the practitioner how proper (from a Yoga point of view) his or her state of mind is.

Conclusions

Muscle fibers are very elastic and in the muscle they are connected with the less elastic connective tissue fibers. This fact is used to explain the loss of flexibility solely as a result of the shortening of the connective tissue in and around the muscles. Such shortening can be caused by lack of movement or by exercising exclusively within less than a full range of motion. But there is more to it than that. Different stretching methods bring about differing results: dynamic stretching improves dynamic flexibility; static stretching improves static flexibility and, to a limited extent, dynamic flexibility. Furthermore the stretching method you choose—ballistic, static relaxed, or isometric—affects the amount of time to achieve results. The possible changes in connective tissues resulting from stretching by any of these methods do not explain all the differences. These differences are most likely the result of the way a given kind of exercise acts upon the nervous system. Muscles are usually long enough to allow for a full range of motion in the joints. It is the nervous control of their tension, however, that has to be reset for the muscles to show their full length. This is why ten minutes of stretching in the morning makes your full range of motion possible later in a day without a warm-up. This is also why repeating movements that do not use a full range of motion in the joints (e.g., bicycling, certain techniques of Olympic weightlifting, pushups) can set the nervous control of length and tension in the muscles at the values repeated most often or most strongly. Stronger stimuli are remembered better. Eastern European coaches will not let their gymnasts ride bicycles, for example, even though they seem to have all the flexibility they need. Strenuous workouts slightly damage the fibers of connective tissue in the muscles. Usually these micro-tears heal in a day or two, but a loss of flexibility is supposedly caused by these fibers healing at a shorter length. To prevent this, some physiologists recommend static stretching after strength workouts. All this sounds very good, but the same gymnasts who are kept from bicycling, run with maximal accelerations to improve their specific endurance. Such running is a strenuous, intensive strength effort for leg muscles, but in running, these muscles work through a full range of motion in the hip and knee joints, and because of that there is no adverse effect on flexibility. If connective tissue were a factor, then stretching after a workout would be enough and these gymnasts could ride bicycles with the same result. The situation with pushups is very similar. If you do a couple of hundred a day, on the floor, so the muscles of your chest, shoulders, and arms contract from a shortened position, no amount of static stretching will make you a baseball pitcher or a javelin thrower.

There are two kinds of stretch receptors, one detecting the magnitude and speed of stretching, the other detecting magnitude only. This explains why flexibility training is speed-specific. Static stretches improve static flexibility and dynamic stretches improve dynamic flexibility, which is why it does not make sense to use static stretches as a warm-up for dynamic action. There is a considerable, but not a complete, transfer from static to dynamic flexibility.

Dynamic stretching by movements similar to the task, for example, leg raises before kicking, lunges before fencing, arm swings before playing tennis, done with gradually increasing range and speed of motion facilitate neural pathways that will be used in the task.

(*Facilitation* means increased excitability of neurons by means of repetitive use or the accumulation of impulses arriving from other neurons.) These movements of gradually increasing similarity in range and speed of motion require muscular contractions increasingly similar to those of the task (kick, fencing attack, serve). These contractions cause arterioles and capillaries in the working muscles to dilate in proportion to the force of contraction. Flexibility improves with an increased flow of blood in stretched muscles. Cutting off the flow of blood to a muscle reduces its elasticity.

Static stretches do not facilitate these pathways, do not prepare the nervous system and blood vessels in muscles for the dynamic task. You even sweat differently when warming up with dynamic actions than when doing static stretches. During dynamic exercises you sweat all over and your sweat is hot. During static stretching you sweat little, mainly on the face. This tells you that static stretching is a poor warm-up.

Flexibility training is also position-specific. Research done by Nicolas Breit (1977), comparing the effects of stretching in the supine and the erect position, shows that:

a) subjects who trained in an erect position tested better in this position than subjects who trained in a supine but tested in an erect position.

b) greater gains were recorded for both groups in a supine test position than in an erect test position. The subjects tested in the erect position had to overcome an extra amount of tension in the muscles they stretched because of the reflexes evoked by standing and bending over.

You can use the postcontractive reflex depression, or inhibition (lower resistance to a stretch), caused by any of the explained mechanisms by contracting a muscle before relaxing and stretching it. This increases the amount of possible stretch. The stretch has to be done within five seconds of relaxation after contraction and preferably in the first second. After reaching a maximal stretch (maximal for you at a given stage of your training), tensing the muscle allows you to hold this position and improve your static strength in it. A strength increase in extreme ranges of motion (occurring after isometric stretching or after you do weight exercises in a full range of motion) seems to be a result of the longitudinal growth of muscle fibers (Fridén 1984) or of resetting the muscle's resting length. Strong muscles tense less than weak ones to support the same load. It means that the strong muscles can be more elongated while still comfortably overcoming resistance.

Coordination and flexibility depend on your emotions too, because of the connection between the cerebellum and the areas of the brain responsible for emotions. Try juggling, balancing, or stretching when you are upset!

The opening caution you read is worth repeating: Mental rigidity—the inability to abandon fixed ideas—is usually accompanied by a low level of physical flexibility.

Recap

The following factors are listed in order of their importance in improving flexibility.

- The greatest and fastest gains are made by resetting the nervous control of muscle tension and length.
- Special strength exercises can stimulate the muscle fibers to grow longer and elongate the connective tissue associated with the muscle.
- Stretching the ligaments and joint capsules and ultimately reshaping joint surfaces takes years and brings about the smallest amount of improvement.

2. How to Stretch

The right stretching method will let you have great flexibility even without a warm-up. Such flexibility is essential for coaches so they can demonstrate a technique immediately when it is needed. A lack of this ability indicates either that the stretching method you use is incorrect, you are chronically fatigued, or both.

Developing great flexibility is one of the easiest tasks in athletic training. It takes little time and effort to reach an exceptional level. Why then do so many people spend hours weekly, year after year, and get such meager results? There are several reasons for it, including the following.

- The wrong exercises
- The wrong timing—doing good exercises, but at the wrong time in a workout
- The wrong choice of training methods, choosing methods that develop other athletic abilities and skills but that interfere with the development of flexibility as well as total athletic development

Applying the principles of methodology you find advocated here in your training will prevent you from making any of the preceding mistakes. These principles are included in the descriptions of stretching methods. If you follow the instructions to the letter, therefore, you cannot go wrong.

In watching or participating in a sport calling for a generation of the maximum force in movement (boxing, track and field—particularly throws and shot put—racquet sports, karate), you have probably noticed that before throwing a punch or hitting a ball, athletes instinctively make a movement in the opposite direction, knowing that this will increase their force. Supposedly, elastic energy is stored during this stretch and recovered during the shortening phase of the movement. When the muscle is relaxed between the stretching and the shortening, however, the prestretch does no good (Hill 1961). This shows the importance of nervous regulation of a muscle's tension. The prestretch stimulates stretch receptors whose impulses raise the activation of motoneurons, thus increasing the muscle's force of contraction. If the connective tissue sheath (fascia), which covers the whole muscle, was the main source of resistance to stretch (and thus of elastic energy) at the ranges of movement permitted in the body, then relaxing the muscle would not make any difference. The muscle encapsulated in its sheath would act like a spring that, once stretched, can only return to its previous length, releasing stored energy no matter when let go.

A muscle works best if contracted from optimal stretch. A longer muscle can exert force on the object (ball, shot, fist) on a longer trajectory, accelerating it more.

There are several methods for improving flexibility. In this book you will find only the safest and most efficient of these. Your choice of method (or combination of methods) depends on your sport and the shape you are in.

Methods of stretching

Dynamic stretching. Dynamic stretching involves moving parts of your body and gradually increasing reach, speed of movement, or both. Perform your exercises (leg raises, arm swings) in sets of eight to twelve repetitions. If after a few sets you feel tired—stop. Tired muscles are less elastic, which causes a decrease in the amplitude of your movements. Do only the number of repetitions that you can do without diminishing your range of motion. More repetitions will only set the nervous regulation of the muscles' length at the level of these less than best repetitions and may cause you to lose some of your flexibility. What you repeat more times or with a greater effort will leave a deeper trace in your memory! After reaching the maximal range of motion in a joint in any direction of movement, you should not do many more repetitions of this movement in a given workout. Even if you can maintain a maximal range of motion over many repetitions, you will set an unnecessarily solid memory of the range of these movements. You will then have to overcome these memories in order to make further progress.

Do not confuse dynamic stretching with ballistic stretching! In ballistic stretches, you use the momentum of a moving body or a limb to forcibly increase the range of motion. In dynamic stretching (as opposed to ballistic stretching) there are no bouncing or jerky movements.

Static active stretching. Static active stretching involves moving your body into a stretch and holding it there through the tension of the muscle-agonists in this movement. The tension of these muscles helps to relax (by reciprocal inhibition) the muscles opposing them, i.e., the muscles that are stretched.

Static passive stretching (relaxed stretching). Static passive stretching involves relaxing your body into a stretch and holding it there by the weight of your body or by some other external force. Slow, relaxed static stretching is useful in relieving spasms occurring in muscles that are healing after an injury. You should not exercise or stretch at all until you have healed sufficiently and you have checked it with your doctor!

Isometric stretching. Using positions similar to those in static passive stretching and adding the strong tensions of stretched muscles, you can cause reflexive relaxations and, subsequently, increases in the stretch. Eventually, when you achieve your maximal (at this stage of training) stretch, you hold the last tension for up to 30 seconds or more. This increases the strength of the muscles in this position. Isometric stretching is the fastest stretching method. Because of the strong and long tensions in this type of stretching, apply it according to the same principles as other strength exercises. You should allow sufficient time for recovery after exercising, depending on your shape, total volume, intensity, and the sequence of efforts. It may be a good idea to use isometric stretching in strength workouts and, on days when recovering from these workouts, use either static relaxed stretching or replace the last, long tension in the isometric stretching by just holding the relaxed muscles in the final stretch.

By combining isometric and static active stretching, you will most quickly develop static forms of flexibility.

In your training, use dynamic stretches right after waking up as your morning stretch, and later, at the beginning of your workout, as a part of a warm-up. Do static stretches after dynamic exercises, preferably in a cool-down. If you need to display static flexibility in the course of your workout or event, then do these exercises at the end of the warm-up.

Early morning stretching

According to Eastern European specialists, if you need to perform movements requiring considerable flexibility with no warm-up, you ought to make the early morning stretch a part of your daily routine. Early morning stretching, which you would do before breakfast, consists of a few sets of arm swings and leg raises to the front, rear, and sides (dynamic stretches). Before doing these raises and swings, warm up all the joints with easy movements. Do not do isometric stretches in the morning. Isometric stretches may be too exhausting for your muscles if you do them twice a day. You must allow a sufficient time for recovery between exercises.

The whole routine can take about 30 minutes for beginners and a few minutes for advanced—after reaching the desired level of flexibility, you will need less work to maintain it. You should not get tired during the morning stretching. The purpose of this stretching is to reset the nervous regulation of the length of your muscles for the rest of the day. Remember: do not work too hard because tired muscles are less elastic and if you overdo it, you will defeat the purpose of this exercise.

Usually, no special cool-down is needed after the early morning stretching. If, in doing a great number of repetitions, you manage to considerably raise your temperature and pulse rate, slow down the pace of the last sets and then spend a minute or two walking. If you have lots of time in the morning, you can also do some relaxed static stretches at the end of your morning stretch.

Stretching in your workout

A properly designed workout plan includes the following parts.

1. The general warm-up, including cardiovascular warm-up and general, dynamic stretching (no static stretches unless you are a gymnast and the routine you practice includes splits and bridges)

2. The specific warm-up, in which movements resemble more closely the actual subject of the workout

3. The main part of the workout, in which you realize your task

4. The cool-down

The whole warm-up should take no more than 30 minutes. About ten minutes of this time is dedicated to stretching. Warming up should involve a gradual increase in the intensity of your exercises. Toward the end of a warm-up, use movements that resemble more closely the techniques of your sport or the task assigned for this workout.

In New York City I have seen people sitting on heaters in order to warm up before a kickboxing workout. Warming up has to prepare all systems of the body in order for you to perform at top efficiency. It has to affect the heart, blood vessels, nervous system, muscles and tendons, and the joints and ligaments—certainly not just one area of the body!

Begin your warm-up with joint rotations, starting either from your toes or your fingers. Make slow circular movements until the joint moves smoothly, then move to the next one. If you start from your fingers, move on to your wrists, followed by your elbows, shoulders and neck. Continue with twisting and bending of your trunk followed by movements in the hips, the knees, the ankles, and finally, the toes. If you start from your toes, the order is reversed. The principles are: from distant joints to proximal (to the center of the body); from one end of the body to the other (top to bottom or vice versa), ending with the part of the body that will be used first in the next exercise. This last principle applies to all parts of a workout.

Next engage in five minutes of aerobic activity such as jogging, shadow boxing or anything having a similar effect on the cardiovascular system. Flexibility improves with an increased blood flow in the muscles.

Follow this with dynamic stretches—leg raises to the front, sides and back, and arm swings, for example. Do leg raises in sets of ten to twelve repetitions per leg. Do arm swings in sets of five to eight repetitions. Do as many sets as it takes to reach your maximum range of motion in any given direction. Usually, for properly conditioned athletes, one set in each direction is enough.

Doing static stretches before a workout that consists of dynamic actions is counterproductive. The goals of the warm-up are: an increased awareness, improved coordination, improved elasticity and contractibility of muscles, and a greater efficiency of the respiratory and cardiovascular systems. Static stretches, isometric or relaxed, just do not fit in here. Isometric tensions will only make you tired and decrease your coordination. Passive, relaxed stretches, on the other hand, have a calming effect and can even make you sleepy.

For several seconds following any type of static stretch your muscles are less responsive to stimulation—your coordination is off (Etnyre and Abraham, 1985). If you try to make a fast, dynamic movement immediately after a static stretch, you may injure the stretched muscles.

After this general warm-up, you can move on to a specific warm-up where the choice of exercises depends on your sport and the subject of the workout. A specific warm-up should blend with the main part of your workout. When the main part is over, it is then time for the cool-down and final stretching. Usually you would only use static stretches here. You can start with the more difficult static active stretches that require a relative "freshness." After you have achieved your maximum reach in these stretches, move on to either isometric or relaxed static stretches, or both, following the isometric stretches with relaxed stretches. Pick only one isometric stretch per muscle group and repeat it two to five times, using as many tensions per repetition (attempt) as it takes to reach the limit of mobility that you have at this stage of your training.

This is the end of your workout. If you do not participate in any sports training, but still want to stretch, just skip the specific warm-up and the main part of workout. Do only the stretches, starting with the dynamic and ending with the static.

If you follow my advice to the letter, and the rest of your athletic training is run rationally, you should be able to display your current level of flexibility within a month without any warm-up. By current level of flexibility, I mean the level you normally display during a workout when you are sufficiently warmed up. Of course, it is still better to warm up before any exercises. Being able to do splits and high kicks does not mean that you are ready to exercise. Warming up lets you perform efficiently during your workout or sports event and speeds up the recovery afterward. Muscles prepared for work do not gather as many of the chemical by-products of effort as the unprepared ones do.

After you attain the required reach of motion, you may reduce the amount of work dedicated to maintaining this flexibility. Much less work is needed to maintain flexibility than to develop it. You will have to increase the amount of "maintenance" stretching as you age, however, to counter the regress of flexibility related to aging.

Flexibility in sports

All sports can be classified according to the character of strength required in them (static, dynamic, explosive); type of effort (aerobic, anaerobic); and other factors. You can also classify sports according to the kind and the level of flexibility needed in them.

There are three kinds of flexibility:

Dynamic—The ability to perform dynamic movements within a full range of motion in the joints.

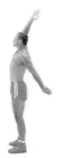 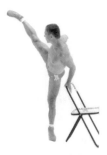

Examples of dynamic flexibility

Static passive—The ability to assume and maintain extended positions using your weight (splits), or using strength not coming from the stretched limbs, such as lifting and holding a leg with your arm or by other external means.

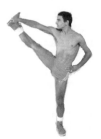

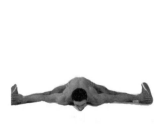

Examples of static passive flexibility

Static active—The ability to assume and maintain extended positions using only the tension of the agonists and synergists while the antagonists are being stretched. One example is lifting the leg and keeping it high without any support.

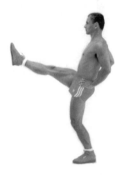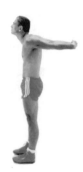

Examples of static active flexibility

The principles of flexibility training are the same in all sports. Only the required level of a given kind of flexibility varies from sport to sport.

The flexibility of an athlete is sufficiently developed when the maximal reach of motion somewhat exceeds the reach required in competition. This difference between an athlete's flexibility and the needs of the sport is called "the flexibility reserve" or "tensility reserve." It allows the athlete to do techniques without excessive tension and prevents injury. Achieving the maximum speed in an exercise is impossible at your extreme ranges of motion, i.e., when you have no "flexibility reserve."

The training of flexibility, as well as of any other motor ability, should proceed in form from general to specific—reflecting the needs of particular sports. In choosing stretches, you should examine your needs and the requirements of your activity. For example, if you are a hurdler, you need mostly a dynamic flexibility of hips, trunk, and shoulders. To increase your range of motion, you need to do dynamic leg raises in all directions, bends and twists of the trunk, and arm swings. You can perfect your technique by doing various dynamic exercises consisting of walking or running over the hurdles. The hurdler's stretch, a static exercise, does not fit into your workout because it strains your knee by twisting it. Simple front and side splits are better for stretching your legs. The explanation that in the hurdler's stretch your position resembles the one assumed while passing the hurdle is pointless. You cannot learn dynamic skills by using static exercises, and vice versa. The technique of running over the hurdles is better developed in motion.

In karate or kickboxing, punches, blows, and kicks should hit their targets with maximum speed. Some targets require the fully stretched muscles of the hitting limb (in the case of kicks, also of the supporting leg). Your nervous system has a way of making sure that a stretch, particularly a sudden one, does not end abruptly, causing a muscle tear. But a gradual slowing down before the moment of contact will spoil the impact. Therefore, you have to train your nervous system (elements of the multineuronal pathway) so you can have maximal speed at the moment of contact even if it is close to the maximal reach of motion in this movement. In the case of kicks, you can learn this skill by using your hand as a target for them. Centers in your brain that regulate coordination and rapid movements know about the hand. They know where it is and that it can stop the kick, so the leg does not have to be slowed down gradually to prevent overstretching.

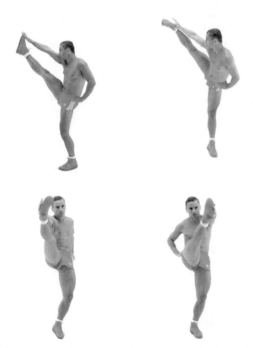

Examples of exercises developing the ability to kick with maximum speed at the ranges of motion required in fighting

You must first develop the ability to move your limbs with moderate speed within a full range of motion in joints in order to do these specific kicking drills. You should start at a lower height to avoid injury from any sudden contraction of rapidly stretched muscles. You can use this exercise only in a warm-up because of the limited variety of kicks that you can practice this way.

Fighters relying on high kicks as their combat techniques should spend a few minutes in the morning on the dynamic stretching of their legs. Starting slowly, they should gradually raise the legs higher. Later they should increase the speed of their movements, perhaps even using the previously described "hand-kicking" drill. Practical experience (North Korean, Soviet bloc's commando units) shows that doing the actual combat kicks in this morning stretch is not necessary to be able to do them later in a day without a warm-up.

Swimmers should have long hamstrings and chest muscles. When doing the breaststroke, if you go up and down in the water instead of moving just under the surface, it means that your chest muscles are too short. In the backstroke this shortness also causes your face to submerge when the arm enters the water, which is when you want to take a breath. In the crawl, short hamstrings pull your feet out of the water and make your legwork inefficient.

Wrestlers and judoka need especially great static strength in extreme ranges of motion to get out of holds and locks. They will best develop this strength by isometric stretching and weightlifting.

Gymnasts and acrobats must display a high degree of development of all kinds of flexibility, with greater emphasis on static active flexibility than in any other sport. Training for and displaying static active flexibility requires good strength in the trunk muscles, especially in the lower back.

You should be careful in choosing your stretches, however, because too much flexibility can be detrimental to your sports performance. For example, in jumping, an excessively loose trunk at the moment of take-off causes a scattering of forces. Olympic weightlifters need to shorten the muscles surrounding the hip and knee joints for the proper execution of lifts. Muscles that are too long let the weightlifter "sink" too deep on his legs while getting under the barbell. This makes it difficult to stand up and complete the lift.

Causes of difficulties in developing flexibility

All elements of athletic training are influenced by each other. For the best results in any one area of training, the methods of developing all the athletic abilities and skills have to be correct.

Here are the most common causes of difficulties in developing an athletic form, flexibility in particular. These are typically faults of training methodology:

The wrong warm-up. Doing static stretches does not sufficiently raise muscle temperature, it does not increase blood flow through muscles, it does not warm up joints, or prepare the athlete for effort.

The wrong training load. Training loads that are too great without enough rest cause chronic fatigue. If you begin your workout still sore after the previous one you are asking for an injury or at least you hamper your further progress.

The wrong sequence of efforts. If you use the wrong sequence of efforts in a workout or in a microcycle, it may double or triple your recovery time. (A microcycle is a set of workouts. It usually lasts one week.)

The wrong methods. Incorrect methods of teaching skills may result in too many repetitions of a given exercise and chronic local fatigue.

The use of partners in stretching

The practice of using partners in stretching is a waste of time, and it is dangerous. The helper is neither stretching nor resting. The danger of using a partner in stretching is obvious. The partner does not feel what you feel. He or she can easily stretch you a bit more than you would like. If you feel pain and let your partner know about it, by the time the partner reacts, it can be too late.

Injury prevention and flexibility

A muscle does not have to be maximally stretched to be torn. Muscle tears are the result of a special combination of a sudden stretch and a contraction at the same time. Great differences in strength between two opposing muscle groups, as well as a strength imbalance of 10% between these same muscle groups on both sides of the body, are the main causes of injuries. Improving the strength of weaker muscles is the best prevention of injuries. A careful analysis of the form of movement may also hold the key to injury prevention. A good technique feels effortless. Eliminate those moments in your technique in which you use the maximal tension of already stretched muscles to counter the fast movement of a relatively big mass. This may lead to tears in the muscles of a supporting leg in kicking, for example. Likewise, if you accelerate suddenly against great resistance, it may lead to a hamstring tear in starting from the starting blocks, for example. Great flexibility alone will not prevent injuries.

If one muscle group, or muscles of one limb or side of the body are more tensed than other muscles you may have a nerve problem or misaligned bones. For example, a twisted pelvis will cause one hamstring to be more tensed than the other. Stretching overly tensed muscles cannot fix the cause of their abnormal tension. In this example, it neither realigns the pelvis nor addresses the cause of this misalignment, which can be neurological or mechanical. While it may make you temporarily feel better, it will not remove a threat of potential injury. This is why static stretching before working out does not prevent injuries.

Children and flexibility training

Preschool children (ages 2 to 5) do not need to dedicate as much time to flexibility exercises as older children and adults, who may have to spend as much as 5-15 minutes per workout on flexibility. Their bodies are so elastic that in the course of natural play they will put their joints through the full range of motion.

From the age of 6 to 10, the mobility of shoulder and hip joints is reduced. To prevent this reduction of mobility, children in this age range must do dynamic stretches for shoulders (arm raises and arm rotations in all directions) and hips (leg raises in all directions). Flexibility of the spine reaches its natural maximum at age 8-9.

Trying to increase the spine's natural range of motion, as well as re-petitive bending and twisting of the spine, causes all sorts of prob-lems—stress fractures to the growth plates of the vertebrae, spondylolysis, spondylolisthesis, and slipped discs—resulting in lifelong back problems. Many gymnasts pay for their spine's great flexibility by wearing body braces and spending the rest of their life in pain.

Avoid static stretches of all kinds (passive, active, isometric) in children's training because excitation dominates over inhibition in a child's nervous system. This means that it is hard for children to stay still, relax, and concentrate properly on feedback from their muscles for periods as long as static stretches require. Isometric stretches require concentration and body consciousness to prop-erly interpret sensations coming from the stretched and strongly tensing muscles so as not to injure them. As with all isometric ex-ercises, isometric stretches may increase the resting tonus of mus-cles, which adversely affects movement coordination—something to be avoided during the limited period in life when one's coordina-tion can be developed. Isometric stretches that start from the standing position, leading to the side split put sideward force on the knees. This force can, with repeated application, deform the joint surfaces of the knees and thus cause loose and knocked knees. Do not do ballistic, isometric, and relaxed stretches before the second stage of adolescence because children's muscles do not resist stretching as much as those of adults and these kinds of stretches cause their ligaments to be stretched. Ballistic stretches, in which you bounce to increase your maximum stretch, are total idiocy in any event. Static active stretches, especially lifting the leg and hold-ing it high without any support, compress the spine and may in-crease lordosis because they bend and twist the spine while the hip flexor (iliopsoas) of that lifted thigh is pulling at the lumbar verte-brae. If you have to do such leg lifts, as might be the case in gym-nastics, for example, you should immediately follow them with exercises and stretches that correct lordosis (pelvic tilts, forward bends).

Age 8 to 11 for girls and 10 to 13 for boys (before the growth spurt) is when you intensify flexibility training because children, by gain-ing mass faster than height, get stronger and more active. In-creased activity without an increased amount and intensity of stretches may reduce their range of motion.

During the growth spurt (11 to 13 for girls and 13 to 15 for boys) height may increase nearly one inch in a month. Muscles and ten-dons do not elongate as quickly as growing bones. Excessive lumbar lordosis, leading to back injuries, results from bones of the spine growing faster than its muscles. Pain in the kneecap, and eventually destruction of its cartilage, is caused by doing too much knee-bending when the quadriceps and hamstrings are tightened by the rapid growth of thigh bones. Stretches should target these muscles that are made tight by the rapid growth of bones, otherwise the child will develop bad posture or get injured. During this first stage of adolescence all bones, ligaments, and muscles are weakened and you should therefore avoid stressing the trunk by many repetitions of bends and twists.

In the second stage of adolescence, after the growth spurt (13-15 for girls, 15 to 19 for boys), you can intensify flexibility training once again and do sport-specific stretches in quality and quantity similar to those for adults—for gymnasts, for example, splits and bridges (static stretches).

* * *

In the following chapters you will find a practical demonstration of principles discussed up until now. The exercises are shown in the sequence that you should use in a workout: from dynamic movements to static ones, gradually moving from a vertical to a horizontal position, each exercise evolving from a previous one. You will find more than the absolutely essential number of stretches for a particular group of muscles. This way, in planning a workout, you have many exercises to choose from and arrange in a methodically correct sequence that suits the subject of the workout. This does not mean that you should do all of them in any of your workouts— one exercise for a given group of muscles is usually enough. Consider facilities where you will work out and what kind of exercises will precede and follow each stretch. You do not want to sit in a puddle to stretch your hamstring or suddenly change position from standing to lying down (or vice versa).

Most photographs in the following chapters show only the final positions of stretches. To start doing any of these stretches you do not have to lean your trunk, spread your legs, or twist your arms as far as these photographs show.

3. Dynamic Stretching

Dynamic flexibility, the ability to perform dynamic movements within a full range of motion in the joints, is best developed by dynamic stretching. This kind of flexibility depends on the ability to combine the relaxing of the extended muscles with the contraction of the moving muscles. Besides perfecting the intermuscular coordination, dynamic stretching improves the elasticity of the muscles and ligaments. The surfaces of joints change in the process of long-term flexibility training.

Fatigue usually reduces dynamic flexibility, so do not do dynamic stretching when your muscles are tired, unless you want to develop a specific endurance and not flexibility. Stretching is most effective when you carry it out daily, two or more times a day. Russian researcher Matvyeyev (1977) cites one experiment: One group of athletes did two sessions of dynamic stretching every day for five days, with thirty repetitions per session. Results for that group were twice as great as for the group that followed a regimen the same in every respect except with a day of rest following each working day. Eight to ten weeks is sufficient to achieve improvement that depends on muscle elasticity. Any further increase of flexibility is insignificant, and it depends on long-term changes of bones and ligaments. Such changes require, not intensive, but rather extensive training, i.e., regular loads over the course of many years.

Dynamic stretches are performed in sets, gradually increasing the amplitude of movements in a set. The number of repetitions per set is between five and twelve. The number needed to reach the maximal amplitude of movement in a joint depends on the mass of muscles moving it—the greater the mass, the more repetitions. A reduction of amplitude is a sign to stop. A well-conditioned athlete can usually make a set of forty or more repetitions at maximal amplitude.

Use dynamic stretches in your early morning stretch and as a part of the general warm-up in a workout. Start your movements slowly, gradually increasing the range and the speed of movements. Do not "throw" your limbs, rather, "lead" or "lift" them, controlling the movement along the entire range. According to Wallis and Logan (1964) the principle of *specific adaptation to imposed demands* in the case of flexibility means that you should stretch at a velocity not less than 75% of the maximal velocity used in your actual skill, a kick, for example.

Dynamic stretches

Neck

Usually you use no special dynamic stretches for the neck. What you have done at the beginning of your warm-up (doing joint rotations) should be enough.

Arms

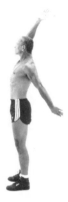

Swing your arms backward at varying angles.

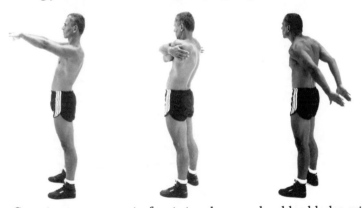

Crossing your arms in front, touch your shoulder blades with your hands, then straighten the arms and touch your hands behind your back.

Legs

Beginners may have to start with a great number of repetitions—four to five sets of ten to twelve repetitions per leg in any given direction, very slowly increasing the height at which the leg is raised. You can switch the leg after each repetition or after a set. After a month or two, you will notice that it takes less repetitions to reach a maximum range of motion. Eventually one set of twelve repetitions in each direction, per leg, will be enough.

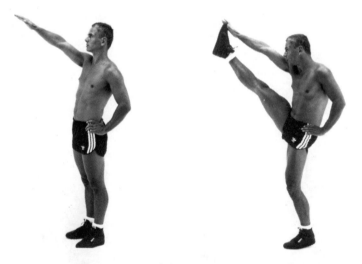

Leg raise to the front. With your hand as a target it is easy to evaluate the progress, maintain good posture (straight trunk) and it can serve as a stop for very dynamic (explosive) leg raises (see page 36). Start as low as feels comfortable. Keep the supporting leg straight, its heel on the ground if possible.

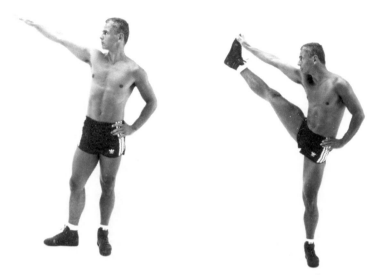

Leg raise to the side. Same as front raise, except the arm is stretched to the side and you raise your leg sideways.

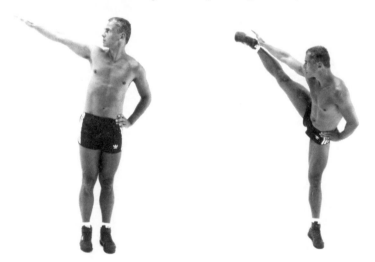

Another form of the side raise. This form is useful for martial artists. The foot of the leg about to be raised points forwards and contact with your palm is made by the side of the foot. Your hips will have a tendency to move to the back and your trunk will lean forward. It is all right, but do not lean forward any more than necessary. Gradually increase the height at which you place your hand, starting at hip level.

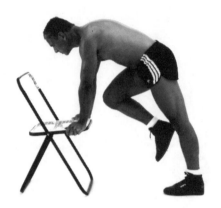

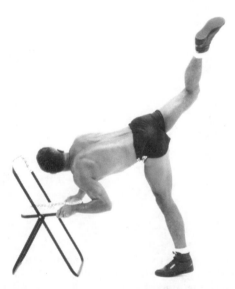

Leg raise to the back. Using any form of support at about your hip height, raise the leg as high as possible. Feel the stretching in front of your thigh.

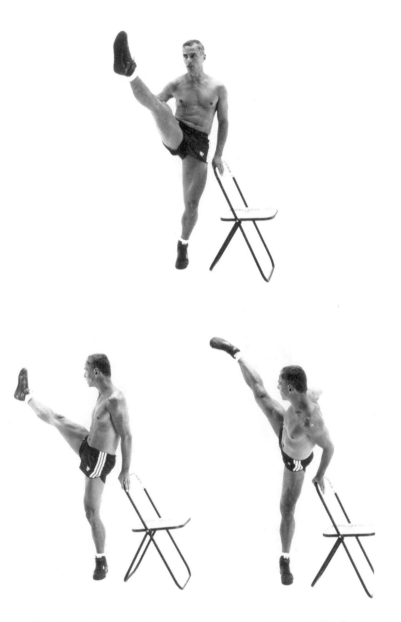

If using a support lets you raise your legs higher to the front and sides—use it.

Trunk

If your sports discipline requires a rapid twisting and bending (with great amplitude) of the trunk, add the following set of exercises to your stretching routines. You can expect to reach full mobility of the trunk (the joints of your vertebral column) in a given direction after 25-30 repetitions of a given exercise.

You can do dynamic stretches for the trunk standing or sitting. A sitting position is better because it isolates the joints of the trunk (vertebral column) from the leg joints. Also, rapid front and side bends in a standing position can become ballistic stretches and injure you.

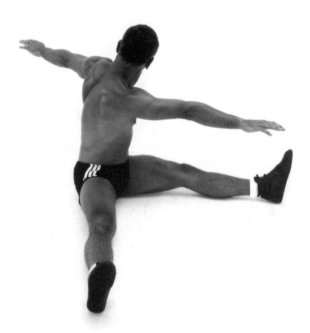

Rotations. Sit down and twist your trunk from side to side. Try to keep your hips and legs immobile.

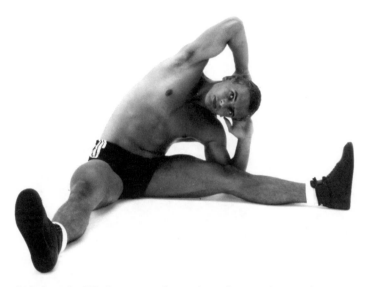

Side bends. While sitting down, lean from side to side.

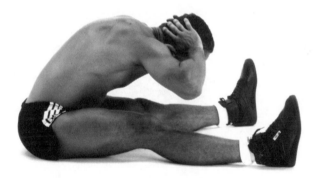

Forward bends. Lean forward from a sitting position. Do not keep your back straight. Let it get round. If you keep it straight, you will stretch your hamstrings instead of your back.

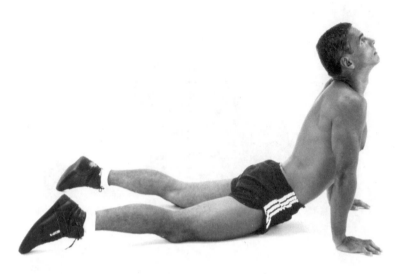

Bends to the back. Lie on your stomach and raise your trunk using your arms and the muscles of the back.

4. Static Active Flexibility Exercises

It is difficult to develop static active flexibility to the level of your dynamic or static passive flexibility. You have to learn how to relax stretched muscles and you have to build up the strength of the muscles opposing them, so that parts of your body can be held in extended positions. Although this kind of flexibility requires isometric tensions to display it, you should also use dynamic strength exercises for its development. In training to hold your leg extended to the side, for example, keep raising and lowering it slowly in one continuous motion. When you can do more than six repetitions, add resistance (ankle weights, pulleys, or rubber bands). After dynamic strength exercises, do a couple of static active exercises, holding the leg up for six seconds or longer, then do static passive flexibility exercises like isometric or relaxed stretches. Your static active flexibility depends on your static passive flexibility and static strength.

If your sport requires dynamic flexibility, let's say for kicking, then you do not need static active flexibility exercises. Holding the leg up is not developing dynamic flexibility nor dynamic strength. It is developing a static active flexibility and static strength required of gymnasts but not something that kickers do need.

Static active flexibility exercises that involve muscles of the back, such as leg extensions and trunk exercises, compress the spine, squeeze intervertebral discs, and may increase lordosis. This compression is especially harmful because it occurs when the spine is already bent, or bent and twisted. To minimize damage, do stretches such as forward bends and pelvic tilts immediately after these exercises. These stretches will relieve spasms of the back muscles and increase the amount of space between vertebrae.

Exercises

In the photographs that follow (pages 52-59), you will see sets of static active flexibility exercises, each set followed by its result.

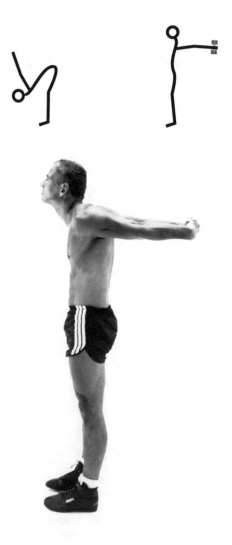

Arm extension to the back.

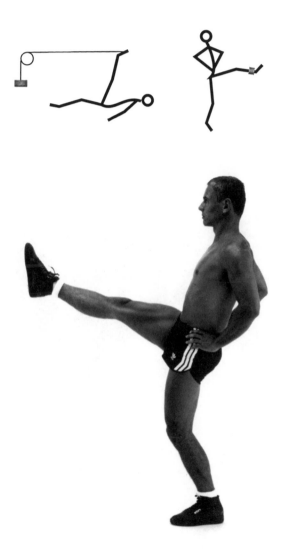

Leg extension to the front.

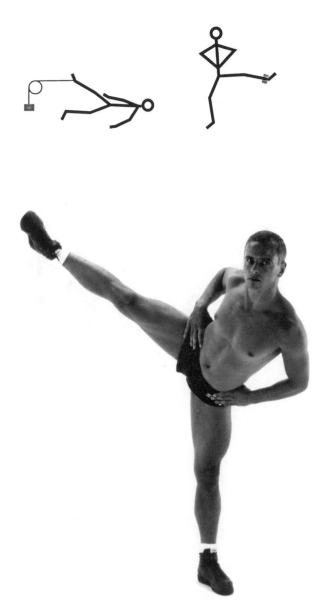

Leg extension to the side.

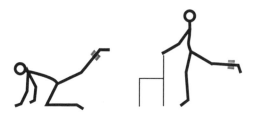

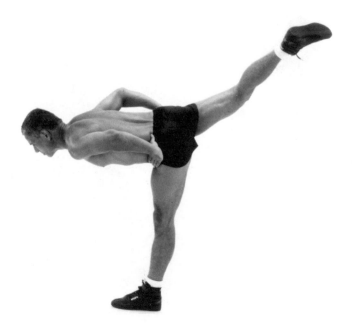

Leg extension to the back.

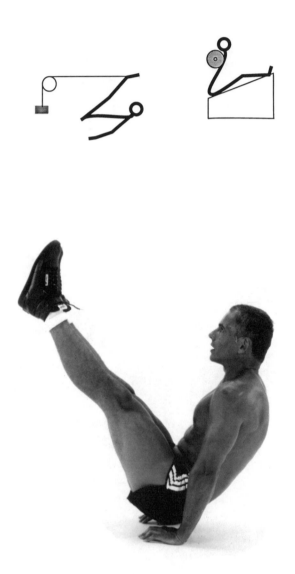

Hamstring and back stretch.

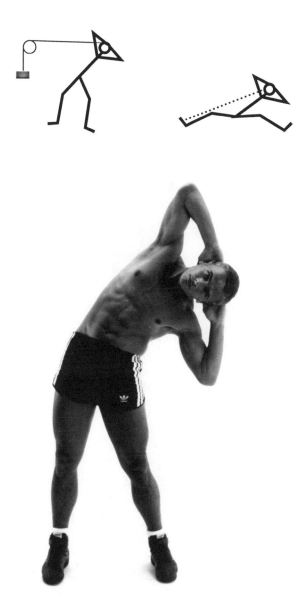

Side bend.

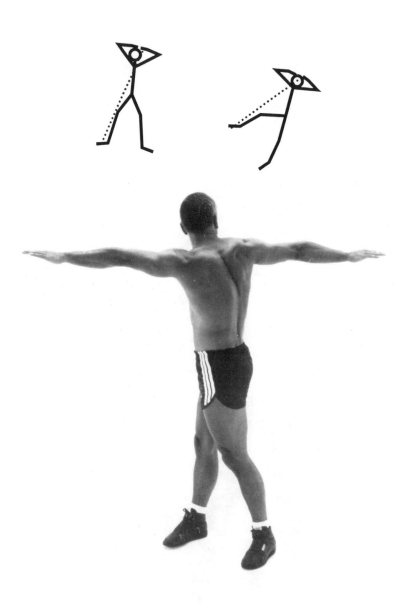

Trunk rotation.

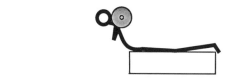

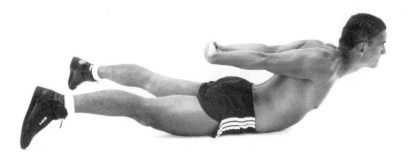

Back extension.

5. Isometric Stretching

In this chapter and in chapter 6, Relaxed Stretching, you will learn how to develop static passive flexibility. Passive flexibility usually exceeds active (static and dynamic) flexibility in the same joint. The greater this difference, the greater the reserve tensility, or flexibility reserve, and the possibility of increasing the amplitude of active movements. This difference diminishes in training as your active flexibility improves. Doing static stretching alone does not guarantee an increase of dynamic flexibility that is proportional to the increase of static flexibility.

Static flexibility may increase when the muscles are somewhat fatigued. This is why static stretching should be done at the end of a workout.

Isometric stretching is the fastest method of developing static passive flexibility. It is not recommended for children and adolescent athletes whose bones are still growing. Your muscles have to be healthy and strong for you to use isometric stretching. If you neglected your strength training, or were doing it incorrectly, the isometric stretches may harm your muscles. In isometric exercises, muscle fibers contract and the connective tissue attached to them is stretched.

When You Are Not Ready for Isometrics

When the connective tissue of a muscle is weak, due to improper strength training, or when it is stretched with too much force, it can become damaged. Depending on the amount of stress and also on the strength of the connective tissue in a given muscle, this damage, at a microscopic level, can announce itself as muscle soreness or it can amount to a complete muscle tear (muscle strain). To make this connective tissue stronger, you should do strength exercises with light resistance and a high number of repetitions. Do these exercises slowly. Make full stops at the beginning and at the end of each movement. You should do at least three sets, with a minimum of 30 reps per set, of exercises for the muscles that are most likely to be overstretched in your sport, or the ones that you intend to stretch isometrically in the near future. Good results are also brought about by doing long single sets of 100 to 200 repetitions. In both cases the weight has to make the last few repetitions "burn."

You should do these high rep exercises at the end of your strength workouts, after the regular heavy weights/low repetition exercises. After these high rep exercises, you should do relaxed stretches for the same muscles.

It is difficult to state for how many months you need to perform the high rep exercises after you have found out that your connective tissue is too weak for isometrics. To find out, you have to periodically test the reaction of your muscles to isometric stretches. If the muscles get sore, it means that the connective tissue is still too weak.

When You Are Ready

Remember the caution in chapter 2: Pick only one isometric stretch per muscle group and repeat it two to five times, using as many tensions per repetition as it takes to reach the limit of mobility that you now have.

Russian researcher Matvyeyev (1977) recommends doing isometric exercises four times a week, ten to fifteen minutes per day, using tensions lasting five to six seconds. The amount of tension should increase gradually and reach a maximum by the third and fourth second. In the particular case of isometric stretching you can hold the last tension, applied at your maximal stretch, much longer, for up to thirty seconds or sometimes even a few minutes. If you are just beginning isometric training, you should start with mild tensions, lasting two to three seconds. Increase the time and the intensity of tension as you progress. Any attempt to develop strength **by isometric exercises only** may lead to a stagnation of strength in only six to eight weeks. To develop exceptional strength as well as flexibility, combine isometric stretches with dynamic strength exercises such as lifting weights, using the same muscles. After a few weeks you may hit a plateau—regulating the tension and length of muscles will stop bringing any improvements in your stretches. Do not worry. Do your exercises concentrating on the strength gains you will achieve. These gains are shown by the increased time you can maintain a position, the amount of weight you can support, or the ability to stand up (slide up, walk up) from your attempts at splits. After some time, when your strength improves, you will notice a great increase in your flexibility.

If, as a result of isometric stretching, or any other exercises, your muscles hurt, reduce the intensity of the exercises or stop working out so you can heal completely. When the pain is gone, if isometrics as stretches or as strength exercises were the cause of the problem, prepare yourself for using them again by doing normal, dynamic strength exercises, gradually increasing resistance. If, for example, stretching your legs by isometric stretches caused pain in any of the leg muscles, stop exercising. Wait till the pain is gone, then try marching, running, running up an incline, climbing stairs, or doing squats. Later you can also do isolated strength exercises using the previously described method (see pages 61-62) of low weight and a high number of repetitions. Do these exercises in such a way as to strengthen the injured muscles. After these exercises and at the end of regular workouts, use relaxed stretches instead of isometric ones until you fully recover. Reintroduce isometrics into your training gradually, adjusting the number and the strength of the tensions, as well as the frequency, in the training week. Make adjustments according to what you feel in your muscles. When everything is all right, you will feel nothing—no pain or soreness.

Several studies have been conducted to determine the number and frequency of the isometric tensions needed for the greatest strength gain, recalling that an increase of strength in isometric stretches means an increased length of muscles. In one study (Hettinger and Müller 1953), subjects with once-per-day sessions, using 66% of maximum contraction, had results equal to subjects using 80% of maximum contraction performed five times per day. Another study (Müller and Röhmert 1963) shows the greatest strength development when using five to ten maximal contractions per day, five days per week. Still other researchers (Fox 1979) report that using maximal contractions every other day is best. Russian researcher Matvyeyev (1977) recommends doing isometrics four times a week, using maximal tension held for five to six seconds, and repeating each exercise three to five times. This is the method I followed because my body responded to it well. You may need a different number, strength, and weekly schedule of isometric tensions. Following is my weekly schedule which suited me well at the time I posed for the photographs in this book. It may be less suitable for someone who works on endurance more often or does more or less weightlifting than I did. This schedule serves only as an illustration of the principle of methodology of training, which can be summed up: "Work on speed or technique before working on strength, work on strength before working on endurance." Violating this principle leads to chronic fatigue, overtraining, or even injuries, and as you remember (see pages 25-26 and 41) fatigued muscles are less flexible than rested ones.

Monday—a technical workout—dedicated to learning or practicing sports techniques— followed by isometric stretching

Tuesday—a strength workout—consisting of strength exercises for the sport—followed by isometric stretching

Wednesday—an endurance workout, that develops endurance for the sport; no static stretching, although if you feel like it you can do relaxed stretches after the workout

Thursday—day off

Friday—a technical workout followed by isometric stretching

Saturday—a speed-strength workout—consisting of strength exercises with stress on speed of movements, followed by isometric stretching

Sunday—day off

This plan assumes that every first day (Monday, Friday) your stretching, as well as your whole workout, will be lighter than on the following day (Tuesday, Saturday). If you "listen" to your body, you will be able to find the combination that works for you. Any muscle soreness or pain is a signal to stop exercises. Do not resume your training if you feel any discomfort or even a trace of pain.

Isometric stretches

There are three methods of doing isometric stretches:

First method: Stretch the muscles (not maximally, though) and wait several seconds until the mechanism regulating their length and tension readjusts, then increase the stretch, wait again, and stretch again. When you cannot stretch any more this way, apply short strong tensions, followed by quick relaxations and immediate stretches (within first second of relaxation) to bring about further increases in muscle length. Hold the last tension for up to 30 seconds.

Second method: Stretch as much as you can, hold this stretched and tensed position until you get muscle spasms, then decrease the stretch, then increase it, tense it, and so on. The last tension should be held for up to five minutes. It makes some people scream.

Third method: This is the one I used to get the results shown in this book. Stretch the muscles nearly to the maximum, then tense for three to five seconds, then relax and preferably within the first second and no later than the fifth second stretch again. Stretch further and further until you cannot increase the stretch. Then hold this last tension for up to 30 seconds. After a minute of rest, repeat the same stretch. Do three to five repetitions of a whole stretch per workout. Use isometric stretches three or four times per week. Gradually increase the time of the last tension to about 30 seconds.

In all these methods, you should concentrate on the strength gains in a stretched position. When you cannot increase the stretch, concentrate on tensing harder or longer, or both. In time it will translate into a greater stretch. To increase the tension of a muscle at any given length—put more weight on it. In splits, not supporting yourself with your arms will help.

No matter which method of isometric stretching you choose, when doing the stretches, breathe as naturally as possible. Natural breathing is not always easy with isometrics, but keep trying.

Neck

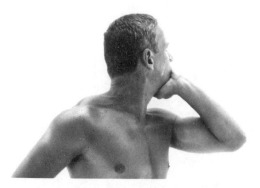

Turn your head to the side, block it with your hand and try turning it back against the resistance of your arm. Relax and turn further in the same direction. Tense again. Hold the last tension for up to 30 seconds. Change sides.

A stretch for muscles of the neck and the upper back: trapezius, sternocleidomastoideus, splenius capitis et cervicis, rectus capitis posterior major, semispinalis capitis et cervicis, obliquus capitis inferior, multifidus cervicis.

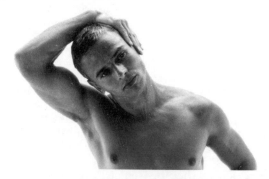

Lean your head toward the shoulder and block it with your arm. Tense the stretched muscles of the neck as if you are trying to straighten your head. Relax and bring it closer to the shoulder. Tense again. Hold the last tension for up to 30 seconds. Change sides.

A stretch for muscles of the neck and the upper back: sternocleidomastoideus, splenius capitis, scalenus anterior, scalenus medius, scalenus posterior, splenius cervicis, longissimus capitis, levator scapulae.

Forearm

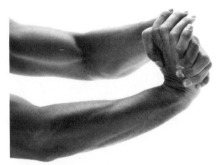

Bend your wrist. Hold your hand, tense, relax, flex more. Hold the last tension for up to 30 seconds. Change hands.

A stretch for the flexors of the hand: flexor carpi radialis, palmaris longus, flexor carpi ulnaris, flexor digitorum sublimis, flexor digitorum profundus.

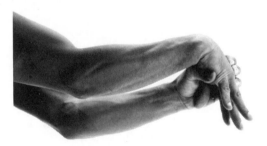

Bend your wrist in the opposite direction. Tense, relax, flex again. Hold the last tension for up to 30 seconds. Change hands.

A stretch for the extensors of the hand: extensor carpi radialis longus, extensor carpi radialis brevis, extensor digitorum communis, extensor carpi ulnaris.

Arms, shoulders, chest

These stretches are for tennis players, swimmers, gymnasts, basketball players, team handball players, golfers, discus and javelin throwers, and hockey players. Students of certain martial arts (Indian muki boxing, wushu, sambo) that require a great mobility of the shoulders will find these exercises useful. Judoka, sambo wrestlers, cyclists, skaters and hockey players can use stretches 1 and 3 as corrective exercises for a rounded back.

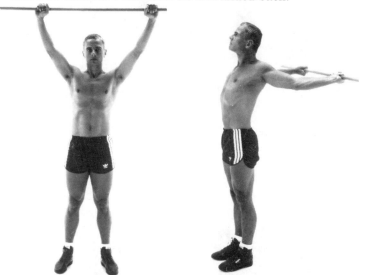

1. Starting from this position, bring the stick to the position behind your back and tense all the stretched muscles. Relax, bringing the stick to the front. Making your grip narrower, bring the stick to the back and tense again. When the grip is so narrow that you cannot lower your arms any more—stop and tense the stretched muscles for up to 30 seconds. This exercise stretches the front of the arms, shoulders and the chest: pronator teres, palmaris longus, brachioradialis, biceps brachii, coracobrachialis, deltoideus, pectoralis major, pectoralis minor, teres major, serratus anterior, subscapularis.

Outside rotation of your arms makes it easier to move them back or up. This is similar to rotating the thighs outside when spreading your legs. Rotating your arm makes the greater tuberosity of the humerus pass behind the acromion (a bone on top of the shoulder) instead of hitting it, so you can move the arm further back or up. Stretch both arms together so the spine movements do not influence the range of movement in the shoulder girdle.

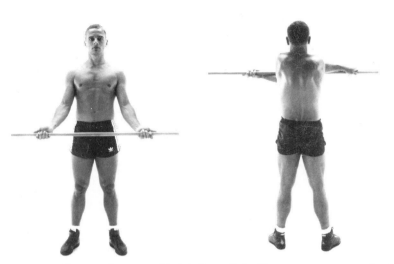

2. Change the grip. Twist the stick. Tense your upper back, shoulders and triceps. Relax. Move your hands further apart on the stick. Twist it again and tense the stretched muscles. Hold the last tension for up to 30 seconds. A stretch for the muscles of the upper back: trapezius, rhomboideus, latissimus dorsi.

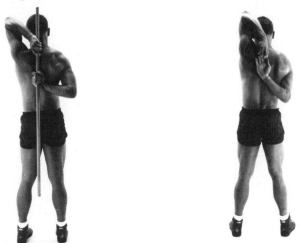

3. Through successive tensions and relaxations, crawl your hands toward each other. Hold the last tension for up to 30 seconds. Switch the position of your hands and repeat the exercise. A stretch for muscles of arms, shoulders, chest and upper back: triceps, anconeus, deltoideus, pectoralis major, latissimus dorsi, teres major, supraspinatus.

Legs

Here are some stretches leading to the side split. They are useful to martial artists, soccer players, skiers, hurdlers, dancers, skaters, gymnasts, judoka, and sambo wrestlers.

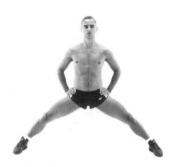

Tense the inside of your thighs as if trying to "pinch" the floor. Relax and spread your legs further. Keep repeating this cycle of tension and relaxation until you cannot lower yourself any more without pain. Hold the last tension for up to 30 seconds. When doing this exercise, do not lean forward and do not support yourself with your arms. Keep your trunk straight. Get out of the stretch without using your arms. A stretch for muscles of the inner thigh: adductor magnus, adductor brevis, adductor longus, gracilis, pectineus.

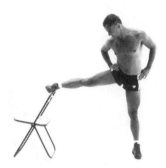

Another version of the previous stretch. Gradually increase the height of the support or the distance from the supporting leg to the support. In the latter case, use something stable and not too high, for example a pile of gymnastic pads, as your support.

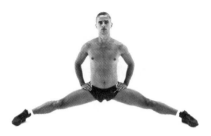

To get from this position to the full side split should take you about one month. At this stage people with weak knees may experience problems. In such cases, strength exercises for the muscles stabilizing the knees will help.

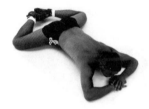

Here is an exercise you can do instead of previous ones should you have any knee problems. The general principle is the same as usual—try "pinching" the floor with your knees and alternate the tensions and relaxations to get your hips as low as possible.

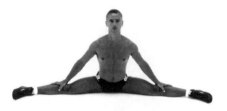

A full side split. Spend 30 seconds or more in this position tensing the inside of your thighs. Try lifting yourself off the floor by the sheer strength of your legs. Eventually you should be able to slide up from the split to a standing position without using your arms. Then you can try a full side split in suspension.

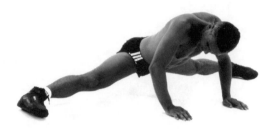

An exercise for a different kind of a side split—a side split with toes pointing upward. Stretches for the muscles described on page 70 and muscles of the buttocks: gluteus medius and gluteus minimus).

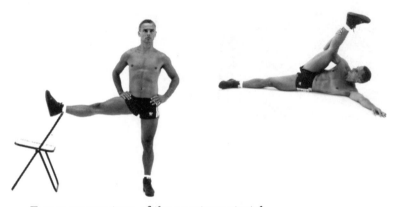

Two more versions of the previous stretch.

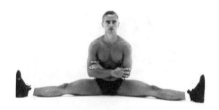

A side split with toes pointing upward.

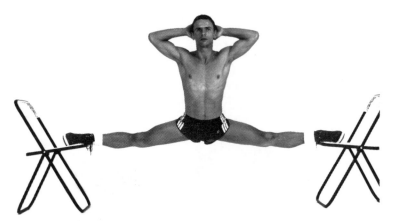

A full side split in suspension. Be careful. A loss of balance may put your muscles out of commission for a year or more. Your first attempts should be done on objects low enough so that you can rest on the floor without tearing the muscles should you happen to lose your balance.

Side splits are not difficult. Anybody with normal range of motion in the joints of the hips and lower back can do them once learning the correct hip-pelvis alignment (Russe, Gerhardt, and King 1972) and with a little strength training of the adductors. Weakness of the adductors is the main obstacle to doing side splits. Weak adductors tense very strongly when you try to spread your legs in the straddle stance. The stronger they are the less tension, pain, and resistance there is while spreading your legs all the way to the floor. Generally the stronger the muscle the fewer motor units are recruited to support any given load (deVries 1980).

Stretches leading to the front split. Important for cyclists, dancers, gymnasts, skaters, skiers, track and field athletes, wrestlers,
judoka, sambo wrestlers, and martial artists.

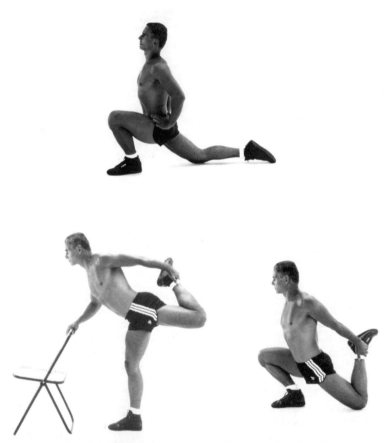

Front of the thigh stretches. Tense the muscles that bring your
thigh forward and straighten your knee. Relax, stretch, tense
again. Hold the last tension for up to 30 seconds. Change sides.
These are the stretches both for the muscles that bring the thigh up
and forward, for example in running, and for the muscles that
straighten the knee: iliacus, psoas major, pectineus, obturatorius
internus, adductor magnus, adductor longus, adductor brevis,
gracilis, rectus femoris, vastus lateralis, vastus medialis, vastus intermedius, sartorius, gluteus minimus, tensor fasciae latae.

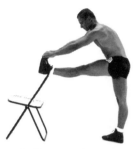
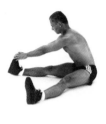

Calf stretches. Grab and pull your toes toward yourself. Point your foot forward against the resistance of your arms. Relax, pull the toes closer to yourself and start pointing the foot forward again. Hold the last tension for up to 30 seconds. Change legs. A stretch for muscles of the calf: gastrocnemius, soleus, plantaris, flexor hallucis longus, tibialis posterior, flexor digitorum longus, peroneus longus, peroneus brevis.

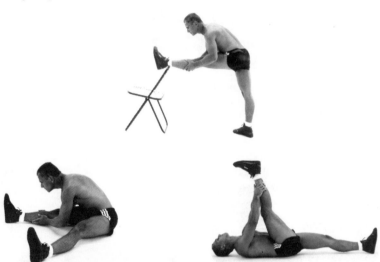

Hamstring stretches. Using one of the positions shown above, stretch your hamstring by increasing the angle between your thighs. Tense the hamstring as if to bring it back down, and then relax it. Pull your leg toward yourself, or if using a support, move the supporting leg further back. Tense again, relax and stretch more. Hold the last tension for up to 30 seconds. Change the leg. A stretch for hamstrings, buttocks and some of the pelvic muscles: biceps femoris, semimembranosus, semitendinosus, adductor magnus, gluteus maximus, gluteus medius, piriformis, obturatorius internus.

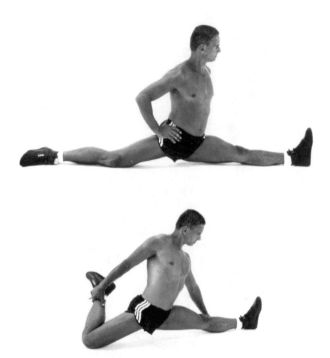

Pinch the floor, tensing the hamstring of your front leg, your quadriceps and the so-called runner's muscles of the rear leg. Relax and lower your hips. Tense again. Hold the last tension for up to 30 seconds. Change sides. A stretch for muscles of the thighs, buttocks and pelvis: iliacus, psoas major, rectus femoris, vastus lateralis, vastus medialis, vastus intermedius, sartorius, adductor magnus, adductor longus, adductor brevis, tensor fasciae latae, obturatorius internus, gracilis, gluteus minimus, pectineus.

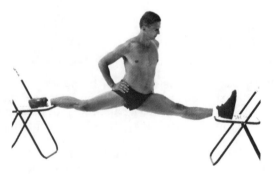

Full front split in suspension.

Trunk

Following are stretches for track and field athletes (throwers), wrestlers, judoka, gymnasts, dancers, and tennis players.

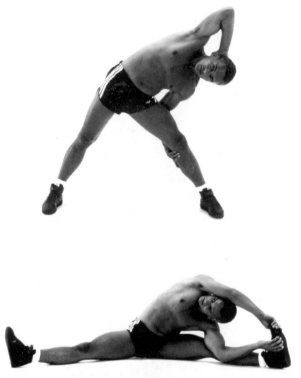

Side bends. Do not twist or lean forward. Move only to the side. Tense the stretched side as if to straighten up, relax and try leaning further to the side. Hold the last tension for up to 30 seconds. Change sides. A stretch for muscles of the side of the abdomen and of the back: quadratus lumborum, longissimus dorsi, iliocostalis, obliquus abdominis externus, obliquus abdominis internus, psoas major.

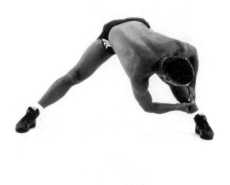

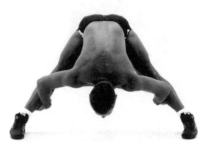

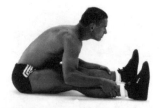

Lower back and hamstring stretches. Grab your legs and tense your back as if trying to straighten up. Relax, lean forward, and tense again. Keep your head straight. Hold the last tension for up to 30 seconds.

Stretches for the muscles of the back, buttocks, hamstrings: longissimus, iliocostalis, multifidus, gluteus maximus, gluteus medius, adductor magnus, biceps femoris, semitendinosus, semimembranosus, piriformis, obturatorius internus, and muscles of the calves.

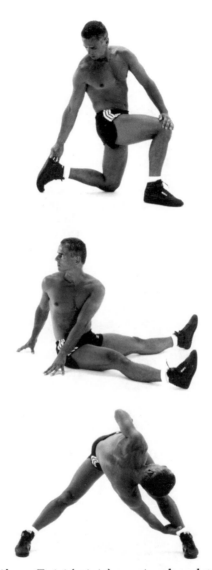

Trunk rotations. Twist (rotate) your trunk and grab your foot or put your hands on the ground. Tense the stretched muscles of your trunk, relax, and twist further. Tense again, relax, stretch and hold the last tension for up to 30 seconds. Change sides. A stretch for muscles of the back and the abdomen: semispinalis, multifidus, muscles rotatores, obliquus abdominis externus, obliquus abdominis internus.

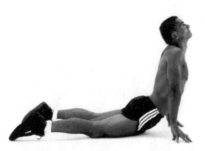

Abdomen stretch. Tense your abdomen as if trying to pull your hips forward and down. Relax, lower your hips, and tense again. Hold the last tension for up to 30 seconds. A stretch for the front of the abdomen, muscles on the front of the spine and the inside of the pelvis: rectus abdominis, obliquus abdominis externus, obliquus abdominis internus, quadratus lumborum, psoas major, psoas minor.

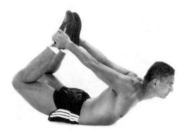

A more intense version of the previous stretch also affecting the front of the thighs. Usually your lower back will get very tense while you do these abdomen stretches. You can even get cramps. To relax the back, do the following "counterstretch," which you can do without tensing.

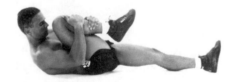

Recap

Isometric stretches are strenuous exercises requiring adequate rest between applications. For best results, supplement them with dynamic strength exercises as described in this chapter on pages 61 and 62. In the workout, all dynamic exercises must precede the isometrics with few exceptions. (One example of an exception: You can include isometric tension before speed-strength actions because it can act as a stimulating factor.) You do the isometric stretches after all the dynamic exercises because of their (isometrics') adverse effect on coordination.

Remember—a partner in stretching can cause an injury. If you need someone's help in doing any stretches, it means that you are not ready for them. It is better to go slowly but steadily.

6. Relaxed Stretching

Relaxed stretches are yet another means of developing static passive flexibility. Although much slower than isometric stretches, relaxed stretches have some advantages over isometrics. They do not cause fatigue and you can do them when you are tired. Problems are unlikely. There are two major drawbacks: your muscular strength in extended positions does not increase as a result of relaxed stretching; and relaxed stretches are very slow. The same person who, in using isometrics, gets into a full side split in 30 seconds without a warm-up may take up to ten minutes of relaxed stretching (with no warm-up) to get to this same level. Within a couple of months of doing relaxed stretches this time gets shorter. Eventually it may take you from one to two minutes to do a full split. (With a good warm-up, of course, you can do it at once.) In your workout, do relaxed stretches last. Do them after isometric stretches or even instead of them. If you have enough time in a day, you can also do them whenever you feel like it, without a warm-up.

In doing these stretches, assume positions that let you relax all your muscles. Some isometric stretches take place in positions designed to tense stretched muscles—e.g., side and front split exercises—by placing your weight on them. In relaxed stretching you want as little weight on your muscles as possible. In splits, lean the body forward and support it with your arms. Relax completely. Think about slowly relaxing all your muscles. Do not think about anything energetic or unpleasant. Relaxing into a stretch, at some point you will feel resistance. Wait in that position patiently and after a while you will notice that you can slide into a new range of stretch. After reaching the greatest possible stretch (greatest at this stage of training), hold it; feel the mild pain in stretched muscles. Get out of the stretch after a minute or two. Do not stay in a stretch until you get muscle spasms. You can repeat the stretch after a minute.

Relaxed stretches

Neck

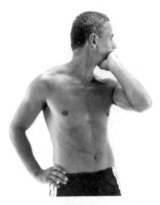

Put your hand on your cheek or your chin. Turn your head to the side. Use your hand to increase the range of motion.

Muscles stretched: trapezius, sternocleidomastoideus, splenius capitis et cervicis, semispinalis capitis et cervicis, rectus capitis posterior major, obliquus capitis inferior, multifidus cervicis.

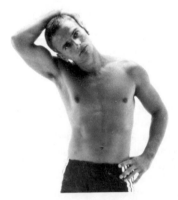

Put your hand on the side of your head. Lean your head toward the shoulder. Use your hand to increase the stretch.

Muscles stretched: sternocleidomastoideus, splenius capitis, scalenus anterior, scalenus posterior, iliocostalis cervicis, splenius cervicis, longissimus capitis, levator scapulae.

Forearm

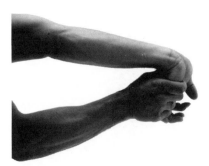

Bend your wrist, using your other hand to increase the stretch.

A stretch for the flexors of the hand: flexor carpi radialis, palmaris longus, flexor carpi ulnaris, flexor digitorum sublimis, flexor digitorum profundus.

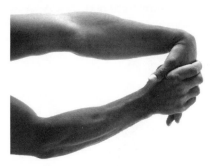

Bend your wrist in the opposite direction, using your other hand to increase the stretch.

A stretch for the extensors of the hand: extensor carpi radialis longus, extensor carpi radialis brevis, extensor digitorum communis, extensor carpi ulnaris.

Arms, shoulders, chest

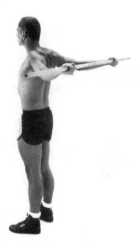

Bring the stick to the position behind your back, using the narrowest grip possible.

A stretch for muscles of the front of the arms, shoulders, and the chest: biceps brachii, pronator teres, palmaris longus, brachioradialis, coracobrachialis, deltoideus, pectoralis major, serratus anterior, subscapularis.

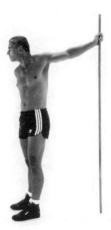

You can stretch the same muscles doing this stretch. Note the outside rotation of the arm. It facilitates moving it up or back.

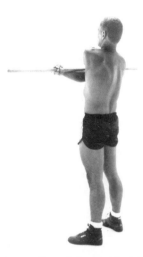

Change your grip on the stick and twist it.

A stretch for muscles of the upper back: trapezius, rhomboideus, latissimus dorsi.

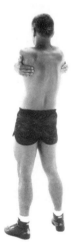

Another form of the upper back stretch.

Crawl your hands on your back as far as you can.

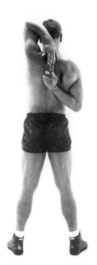 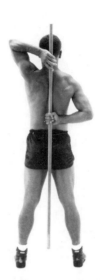

Grab your hands behind your back. If you cannot, use a piece of rope or a stick to crawl your hands toward each other. In turns, pull down the upper hand, then pull up the lower hand to feel a good stretch.

Muscles stretched: triceps, anconeus, deltoideus, pectoralis, latissimus dorsi, teres major, supraspinatus.

Remember that stretching both your arms together eliminates the influence of movement in the spine on the range of motion in your shoulder girdle.

Legs

Exercises leading to the side split.

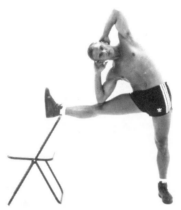

Place your leg on any support. Either lean toward this leg or move the other leg away from the support.

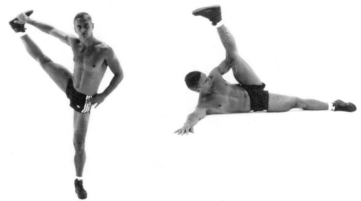

You can also lift your leg with your hand.

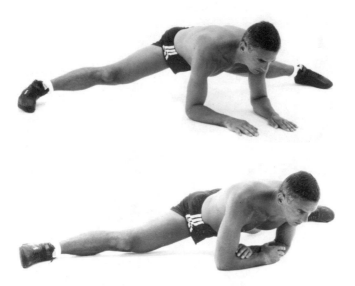

Stretch the muscles of both your inner thighs in this position. Shift your weight between your legs and arms to get the best stretch. When your legs tense, help them relax by putting most of your weight on your arms. When the legs relax, slide into a greater stretch by shifting your weight back.

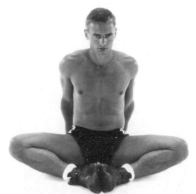

One more, even milder inner thigh stretch. Sit down, bend your knees and pull your feet together. Now, lower the thighs using only the strength of the muscles that abduct and rotate them externally. Do not push with your hands.

Stretches for muscles of the inner thigh: adductor magnus, adductor brevis, adductor longus, gracilis, pectineus.

Exercises leading to the front split.

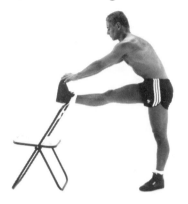
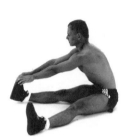

Calf stretches. Pull your toes toward yourself. Feel the stretching in the muscles of the calf: gastrocnemius, soleus, plantaris, flexor hallucis longus, tibialis posterior, flexor digitorum longus, peroneus longus, peroneus brevis.

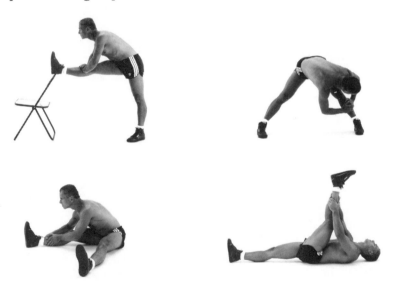

Hamstring stretches. Using any of the above shown positions, stretch your hamstrings.

Muscles   stretched: biceps   femoris,   semimembranosus, semitendinosus, adductor magnus, gluteus maximus, gluteus medius, piriformis, obturatorius internus.

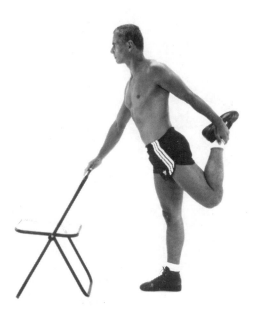

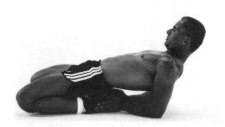

Quadriceps stretches. These are stretches for the muscles of the front of the thigh and the so-called runner's muscles originating inside the pelvis and in front of the spine: iliacus, psoas major, rectus femoris, vastus lateralis, vastus medialis, vastus intermedius, sartorius, adductor longus, adductor brevis, tensor fasciae latae, obturatorius internus, adductor magnus, gracilis, gluteus minimus, pectineus.

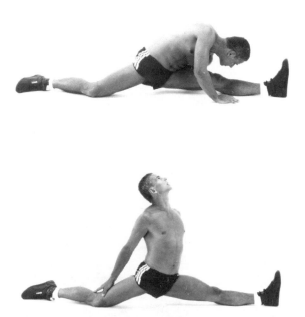

Sit in the split. Lean your trunk forward and backward to stretch all the muscles of the thigh, buttocks, and pelvis.

Muscles stretched: iliacus, psoas major, rectus femoris, vastus lateralis, vastus medialis, vastus intermedius, sartorius, adductor magnus, adductor longus, adductor brevis, tensor fasciae latae, obturatorius internus, gracilis, gluteus maximus, gluteus medius, gluteus minimus, pectineus, biceps femoris, semimembranosus, semitendinosus, piriformis.

Trunk

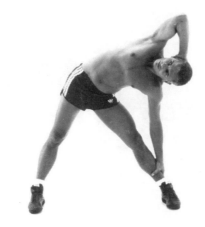

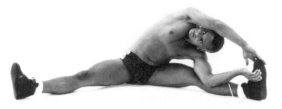

Side bends. Bend your trunk to the side. Do not twist or lean your trunk forward.

A stretch for the muscles of the back and the side of the abdomen: quadratus lumborum, longissimus dorsi, iliocostalis, obliquus abdominis internus, obliquus abdominis externus, psoas major.

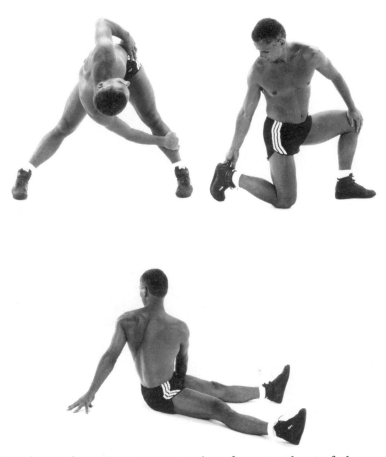

Trunk rotations. Rotate your trunk as far as it takes to feel a mild stretch. You can increase the stretch and help yourself keep it by putting your hand on your leg or on the floor.

Muscles stretched: obliquus abdominis externus, obliquus abdominis internus, semispinalis, multifidus, muscles rotatores.

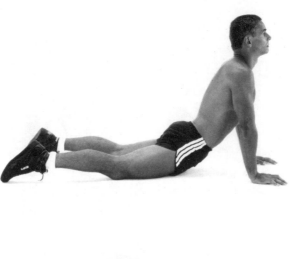

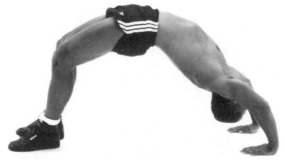

Abdomen stretches. Stretches for the front of your abdomen and the muscles on the front of the spine and the inside of the pelvis: rectus abdominis, obliquus abdominis externus, obliquus abdominis internus, quadratus lumborum, psoas major, psoas minor.

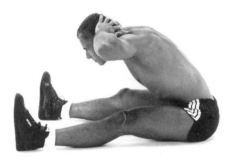

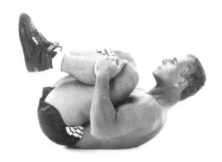

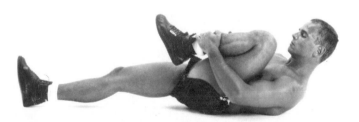

Lower back stretch. Stretch as much as it takes to relax the muscles of the back and not stretch its ligaments. Stretching the ligaments of the back weakens it. This is why you will not see here a relaxed stretch for the back in a standing position. The weight of the upper body hanging on your relaxed spine can stretch its ligaments. To feel a stretching in the muscles of your back, arch it. Keeping your back straight stretches your hamstring.

Muscles stretched: longissimus dorsi, iliocostalis, multifidus.

7. Sample Workout Plans

Here you get examples of how to choose exercises depending on the task of your workout and when to do them in the course of the workout. You will find several sport disciplines listed. Each is represented by one workout with the task common for that discipline. These are just examples and not prescriptions. In a professionally run training process, no workout is the same. Each workout has either a different task or the task is realized by a different means every time. Different tasks and different means of their realization are assigned to workouts depending on the age, class, and condition of the athletes. In planning a workout the coach has to take into consideration the workouts done thus far, the next tasks that need to be done, when the athletes need their form to peak, and much more. To put it simply: your skill level and condition change from workout to workout, and so do your exercise needs.

In the following examples you will see only the flexibility exercises related to the task of the workout. The exercises of the main part of the workout are not shown.

Discipline: Track and Field—Hurdles. Task of the workout: The technique of passing the hurdles; no work on the start from the blocks or on the finish

General warm-up

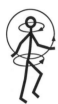   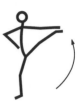

Jogging with rotations of the joints   March with knee raises   March with leg raises to the front   March with leg raises to the side

Specific warm-up

March with passing hurdles

Main part

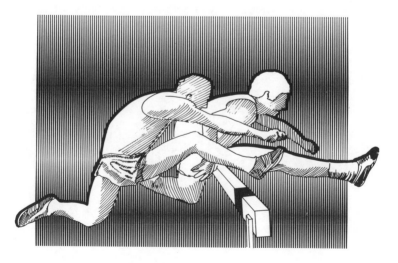

Cool-down

Jogging   March with lunges

Isometric stretches

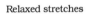

Relaxed stretches   March

Discipline: Gymnastics. Task of the workout: The development of flexibility and the perfection of the handstand (a task usually realized with children nine to ten years old)

General warm-up

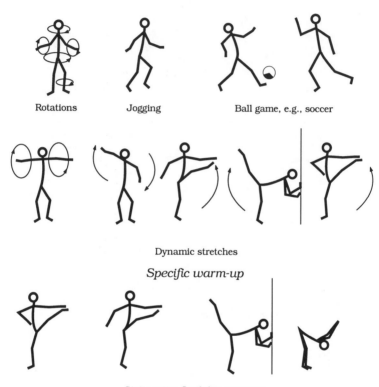

Rotations   Jogging   Ball game, e.g., soccer

Dynamic stretches

Specific warm-up

Static active flexibility exercises

Relaxed stretches

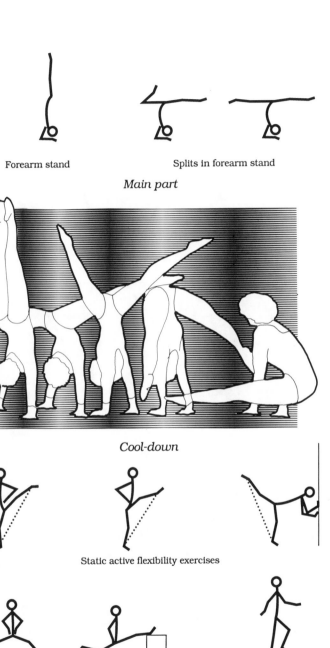

Forearm stand   Splits in forearm stand

Main part

Cool-down

Static active flexibility exercises

Isometric stretches   March

Discipline: Kickboxing. Task of the workout: The high round-house kick

General warm-up

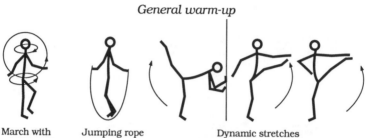

March with   Jumping rope   Dynamic stretches
rotations of
the joints

Specific warm-up

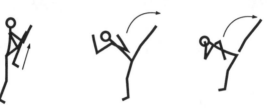

Knee kicks   Roundhouse kicks

Main part

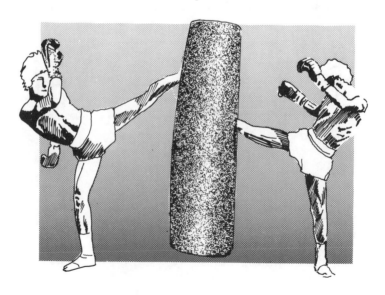

Cool-down

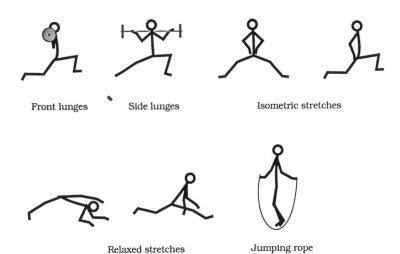

Front lunges   Side lunges   Isometric stretches

Relaxed stretches   Jumping rope

Discipline: Judo. Task of the workout: Teaching O-Soto-Gari (big outside sweep)

General warm-up

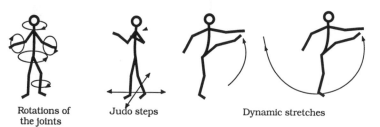

Rotations of   Judo steps   Dynamic stretches
the joints

Specific warm-up and main part of the workout

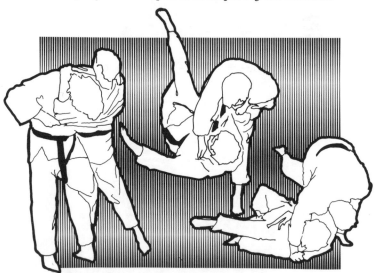

Cool-down

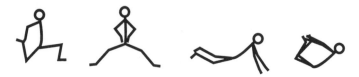

Isometric stretches

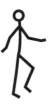

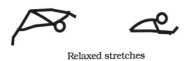

Relaxed stretches

March

Discipline: Bodybuilding. Task of the workout: Developing strength in the upper back, chest, forearms and lower legs

General warm-up

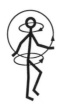
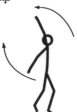

March with rotations of the joints   Dynamic stretches

Specific warm-up and main part of the workout

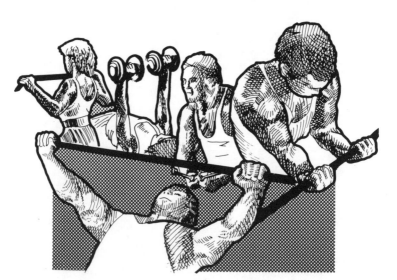

Cool-down

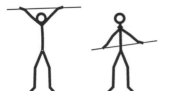

Isometric stretches

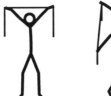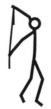

Relaxed stretches

Discipline: Swimming. Task of the workout: Speed in the butterfly stroke

General warm-up

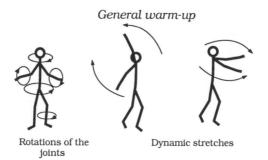

Rotations of the   Dynamic stretches
joints

Specific warm-up, main part and most of the cool-down in the pool

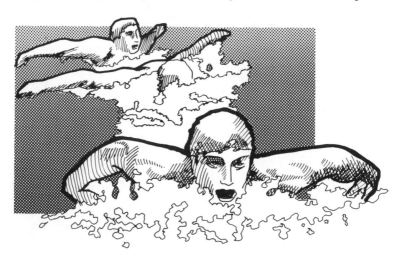

Cool-down

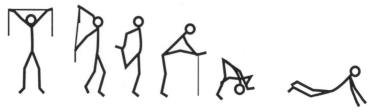

Relaxed stretches

8. Questions and Answers on Stretching

These are typical questions from readers of this book. Among them may be just the type that you want to ask. Study the answers, and perhaps you will be able to apply them to your situation.

Question: Is it truly possible to produce a permanent, instantly accessible flexibility that requires no warm-up or any other preparation?

Answer: Yes. Otherwise what is the point of practicing combat techniques such as high kicks if they require a warm-up? I personally know many athletes, some of them active soldiers, who can display much greater flexibility without a warm-up than what I show in this book. Of course, I can do everything that you see in this book also without a warm-up. If your coach or instructor cannot teach you how to have such flexibility then it tells you something about his or her knowledge of human physiology and the methodology of sports training.

Question: How do you get on those chairs?

Answer: One way is to stand on them when they are close to each other and then spread your legs with the chairs. Another way is to place the chairs so they are as far apart as your feet in a split and then do a handstand between them, lower your legs onto the chairs and push off the floor with your hands to assume the final position. When trying to learn this skill, you should start on two books or small blocks of wood.

Question: Can you tell me how to get strong enough to be able to support someone while I sit in a suspended split between chairs?

Answer: I do not advise you to try lifting or holding anybody while in a split (as shown in my advertisements).

I did it to prove the superiority of my method of strength and flexibility training and had to rest for a week afterward (maybe because we made so many attempts—it took 15 attempts, each 10-20 seconds). The type and amount of strength needed for holding a model on the thigh in a split has no application in sports. The exercises leading to this result are the same as shown on the video *Secrets of Stretching.*

Question: How often should suspended splits be tried, and how do you maintain your strength and flexibility once you have achieved a suspended split?

Answer: Every time you can lift yourself off the floor while sitting in a split you are proving that you have enough strength to do a suspended split. I do not see any reason for most athletes ever to try an actual suspended split. I did it to catch your attention, but as far as strengthening legs goes there are many better and safer exercises.

I maintain my strength by first extending the time (usually up to 30 seconds) of holding a certain weight while I am in a split, then by adding more weight and reducing the time, and again increasing the time with the new weight. Thirty seconds with 100 pounds in your hands while sitting in a split gets really long.

Question: How old is the man demonstrating splits with a girl sitting on his thigh?

Answer: Thirty-five at the time this picture was taken.

Question: How old were the guys in the picture [showing three STADION instructors hanging in side splits between chairs] when they started doing their stretching exercises?

Answer: The first one—Tom Kurz, at 22; the second—Marek Drozdzowski, at 12; the third—Richard Korczynski, at 20.

Question: I wonder about the results of your method in people past thirty years of age. I started taekwondo in my late thirties and currently I am forty-two years old. I would like to know if it is possible for me to do the splits without injuring myself?

Answer: As long as your muscles are responsive to strength training they are also responsive to stretching. We have plenty of testimonials from people past their thirties saying and showing that they just achieved a full side split.

Question: What is the difference between suspended splits with toes pointing forward and with toes pointing upward?

Answer: The split with toes pointing forward stresses adductors and does not require great mobility (outside rotation) of the hip joint. The split with toes pointing upward stresses your hamstrings and you cannot do it if you do not have great outside rotation of the hip joint.

Question: On page 72 you show a side split with toes pointing up. Why do you not describe how to gradually stretch into this position?

Answer: Because you can stretch for this split the same as for the one with toes pointing forward. Alignment of hips and thighs in both splits is the same, as is explained on page 16.

Question: In chapter 5, "Isometric Stretching," the word *tense* is used to describe the method for performing the stretches. Do you mean tighten up your muscles?

Answer: Yes, I mean tighten up your muscles as if to flex the stretched limb or counteract the stretching.

Question: How many times per week should one do isometric stretches? Is it the same as with lifting weights, in which case each body part is exercised 2 or 3 times per week?

Answer: Both isometrics and lifting weights are strength exercises. They both should be done during the same workout (strength workout). More information on this and on related subjects is in the book *Science of Sports Training.*

Question: Can a stretching machine be used to aid stretching?

Answer: There is no need for using stretching machines. In relaxed stretches you can as easily relax into a stretch on a smooth floor. In isometric stretches, a machine will make it more difficult for you to tense your muscles because it prevents the weight of your body from pressing on your legs and thus forcing them to tense more. The harder you tense in isometric stretches the greater is the following relaxation and the resulting stretch.

Question: I have difficulty deciding what exercises to do and the proper sequence of exercises to achieve maximum results. What help can you offer me?

Answer: I assume that by exercises you mean stretches. If not, if you mean other exercises, then *Science of Sports Training* will answer your question. Concerning stretches—do dynamic stretches similar to the movements in your sport. Do those isometric stretches that resemble positions at which your range of motion is less than required in your sport. For example, stretches 1 and 3 on pages 68 and 69 would help for baseball pitchers. Gymnasts or kickboxers may pick any stretch from pages 70-72, plus any stretch from page 74 and any hamstring stretch from page 75. Stretches you do for the front of the thigh and hamstring you can later replace with front splits (page 76) as your flexibility improves. You can do relaxed stretches similar to your isometric stretches or whichever ones stretch your tensed muscles.

The proper sequence of stretches in a workout is: dynamic, static active, isometric, relaxed. You do not have to do all these types of stretches in a workout. You can skip the ones that you do not need but do not alter the order.

Question: How should I introduce this method into my martial arts workout?

Answer: Do dynamic stretches at the beginning of your workout, after the aerobic part of the warm-up. Then do your techniques or sparring. At the end of the workout, do your strength or conditioning exercises, then do isometric stretches and follow them with relaxed stretches. If you do your strength exercises in a separate workout, then do dynamic stretches in the warm-up, and isometric stretches at the end of that workout. Do relaxed stretches in the cool-down of any workout, either after isometric stretches or instead of them. I do not recommend doing isometric stretches every day. Two to four times per week, depending on the reaction of your muscles, is enough.

Question: How many static stretches should I do in my workout?

Answer: Pick one or two isometric stretches—for example one for adductors and one for hamstrings—and one or two relaxed stretches for the same muscles. Do as many sets of isometric stretches as you need to reach your current maximum range of motion, but do not force yourself if your muscles are tired and stale. Three to five sets per stretch should be enough. Then, after isometric stretches, you can do relaxed stretches for one or two minutes each.

Question: Is it safe to do six or seven sets of isometric stretches in one workout?

Answer: It is safe as long as you do not feel pain while exercising. I would not be surprised, though, if you were so sore after this workout that you would have to rest your legs for a few days. In isometric stretches, as with most strength exercises, it is neither safe nor necessary to completely exhaust the muscles.

Question: How do my isometric stretches change once I am able to lift myself up from the floor while in a split?

Answer: If you want to further increase the strength of your hamstrings and adductors, you can try to increase their tension by holding weights in your hands, or put a weighted belt on, or press or pull against some immovable object.

Question: To increase resistance and thus the tension of my muscles in a split, I hold a long stick and press it against the ceiling while trying to lift myself from the split. What do you think about such a way of increasing resistance?

Answer: Your idea of using a long stick that touches the ceiling to add resistance has an advantage over my method of holding weights—it allows you to apply resistance at precise angles and in moments that you choose. It also seems safer than holding weights because you can apply tension gradually and release it faster than you can throw down the dumbbells. The drawback, comparing the use of the stick to dumbbells, is that you do not know precisely how much resistance you apply.

Question: You say that in an attempt to develop exceptional strength and flexibility one should combine isometric stretches with dynamic strength exercises such as lifting weights. If lifting weights, what exercises do you recommend?

Answer: Squats, lunges, step-ups, deadlifts, good mornings, leg extensions, leg flexions.

Question: The mornings are the best time of the day for my karate workouts. My question is: Can I do isometric stretches at the end of those morning karate workouts or do I have to do isometric stretches in the evening?

Answer: It depends on your objective. If having great flexibility during the day without a warm-up is not your objective, then you can do isometrics in the morning. If you want to be flexible during the day after your morning karate workout, you can postpone isometrics as well as other strenuous strength exercises until late afternoon or evening. Just make sure that you warm up well. You have to monitor your progress and if your strength and flexibility keep improving while you do isometrics in the morning workouts, then it is fine to do them then.

Question: I am sixteen years old. Is it possible to do splits at my age?

Answer: Yes, it is possible, but unless you are past the growth spurt it is safer to refrain from the isometric stretches that are the quickest way to achieving splits.

Question: My instructor makes the class do static stretches before a workout comprised of kicking. Is it okay to do static stretches before kicking?

Answer: I would not do these stretches—see pages 24, 25, and 31 for a detailed explanation.

Question: Do static stretches have to be part of a workout, or can I do them by themselves?

Answer: It is better to do them at the end of the workout when your muscles are well warmed up. This applies particularly to isometric stretches. You can do relaxed stretches by themselves, but please do them slowly so you do not hurt unprepared muscles.

Question: Is it okay to perform relaxed stretches after I have already cooled down from a workout?

Answer: Yes, but do them slowly and realize that it will be more difficult than when you are warmed up.

Question: After reading chapter 1, "Theory," I tried to determine my flexibility potential for a side split. I can't tilt the pelvis forward *and* rotate my thighs outward. If I can't do that, then do I have a hip structure problem or is it just that my hip ligaments are very tight? What should I do to overcome this problem?

Answer: I think that you have misunderstood the side split test. It seems that you tried to simultaneously tilt your pelvis forward and rotate your thighs outward. That must be really difficult. I tried it and I could not do it either.

The test does not require tilting your pelvis forward—only rotating your thigh and raising it at the hip level. Please read the book carefully and do the test *as shown* on page 16.

Question: What determines the speed of progress in stretching?

Answer: The speed of progress in stretching depends on your initial strength level and initial flexibility level, and on how rational your total training program is. Normally it takes well under a year to develop the ability to perform splits. I would like to take this opportunity to give you one essential training tip: Consider isometric stretches to be *strength* exercises and apply them as such. Use sufficient rest between workouts. Do not do more exercises than you need, i.e., do not do more than two isometric stretches per workout (you may do a few repetitions of a stretch but do not do many various stretches). Do not overwork any group of muscles.

Question: I am a 36-year-old martial artist who has been practicing about eight years. I have been an athlete all my life, and have used many strength and stretching techniques. Your methods have been the most effective for me. After using your methods I find my kicks are stronger than before and I can "recall" my maximum stretch with very little warm-up. The problem I seem to have now is that I have reached a "sticking point" in my side splits and can't get further down than what you show in the top photo on page 71. I maintain my body in the upright position when doing side splits and don't use my hands for balance. I usually do three to five sets holding each tension for 20-30 seconds and concentrate on strength gains as you suggest. I have reread your book several times and it appears to me that I'm using your methods correctly. Why, then, can't I progress beyond the "sticking point"?

Answer: The cause of a "sticking point" may any one of the following:

a) lack of strength of all muscles of the thigh (try low squats, one-legged squats, dead lifts, adductor flies, adductor pull-downs);

b) not tilting hips forward while spreading legs in a split;

c) not getting enough rest between workouts (doing more than two strength workouts per week); or

d) doing isometric exercises too often (2-4 times per week is enough).

Question: I have been using your method for two years and I still can't do the side split. Perhaps I am doing something wrong. I train in the evening. I begin with leg raises to the front, back, and sides (12 repetitions per leg and per direction). Then I hold my front kick position for 10 seconds each leg, then side kick position for 10 seconds each leg (static active flexibility exercises). I repeat the whole thing three times. Could you tell me what my mistakes are and the quickest method for me to achieve the side split?

Answer: Your inability to perform a side split may be caused by:

a) lack of strength in your adductors (inner thigh muscles); and

b) not tilting your hips to the rear while sliding into a split (see pages 16 and 17). Also I noticed that you did not mention performing dynamic stretches (leg raises) in the morning. In your evening workout you can skip the leg holding (static active flexibility exercises) to save time and energy for isometric stretches.

Question: I have used your method for about a month, and although my flexibility has increased, I still start my splits from the same height above the floor. I can spread my legs further but the starting position is the same. Will this change?

Answer: Your starting position for the split will get lower when the strength of your legs increases more.

Question: What are the possible causes of inconsistency in flexibility? My own flexibility is often very inconsistent. From week to week, sometimes even day to day, it varies anywhere from near split to that of a rank beginner. I seem to have the worst flexibility and most soreness a day or two after a particularly good kick workout in which my legs were very limber and relatively free of pain.

Answer: You say "relatively free of pain." Does this mean that most of the time your legs hurt? If so, no wonder your flexibility suffers—tired or hurt muscles are less flexible than rested and healthy ones. From what you say it seems that the inconsistency in the level of flexibility you display is caused by irrational training. You do not have enough strength and muscular endurance for your kicking workouts and so after such a workout you are sore and inflexible.

Question: I'd like to ask you why after achieving a great stretch my muscles seem to tighten again. For example, I get myself into a full lotus, and then for a whole week after I can't get even close to it.

Answer: I think that there are two possible reasons for your problem:

a) You may be overstretching your muscles.

b) You may be overworking them with other exercises.

Carefully following the advice in this book and in the video *Secrets of Stretching* should solve your problems.

Question: I am 28 years old, reasonably fit, hold a black belt in taekwondo, and have used your method of stretching for about three months. I work shift work, and as a result can only attend formal training two times a week every second week. My taekwondo workouts are pressed for time and so the warm-up and stretching is far too quick and not in the correct sequence that you recommend. I have been doing taekwondo for seven years now and the stretching done in class has never really improved my flexibility. I find that if I skip training in any form for about a week or two I am *more* flexible but then get sore later after resuming my taekwondo workout. Even when following your guide, after a taekwondo session I am too sore and stiff (in my hamstrings) to work out daily by your method. What is the cause of my soreness and lack of progress in flexibility?

Answer: There are two possible causes of your lack of progress in flexibility development:

a) The taekwondo workouts are run by a possibly good fighter but a lousy coach. (You said that exercises are not done in the correct sequence.)

b) Your muscles are too weak for these workouts. Soreness after a workout indicates it.

My advice is to stop attending taekwondo workouts and gradually bring your flexibility, strength, and endurance to such a level that after a few month you can safely return to taekwondo.

Your training has to be systematic, with gradually increasing workloads. Please follow the advice from this book or the video *Secrets of Stretching*.

Question: Within the two months that I have been following your program my flexibility has improved a great deal. In the side split I am lower than I have ever been in all my [five] years of [karate] training. Upon receiving your videotape I stopped going to karate because I wanted to concentrate only on my splits. I did not want to go through the pain of stretching in class. In other words I did not want to mix the two different styles of stretching. Now that my flexibility has improved I started to attend karate workouts again and my joints are sore. When I kick I feel some pain, even when the kick is below the belt. Is this normal? I know for a fact that my joints are more tight than most people's. Is it possible to change this?

Answer: Regarding your question on the cause of joint pain or soreness after returning to karate training, I cannot give you a definite answer because I do not know enough about you and your training. Some of the possible causes may be:

a) poor kicking technique (bad body alignment, not leaning back in roundhouse and side kicks);

b) inadequate strength training (as shown and explained in the video *Secrets of Stretching*);

c) not enough (or wrong) dynamic stretching in the morning and later in the day (it has to be done twice a day, on workout days during your warm-up);

d) doing too much too soon; and

e) abnormal or injured joints (consult your doctor).

Question: Yesterday I did a workout with a lot of kicking and today my hamstrings are sore. Is this due to my muscles not being strong enough? Or not flexible enough? What should I do to stop my hamstrings from getting sore? They do not get sore after lifting weights—only after kicking.

Answer: Kick less and lift more. Make sure that you move through the full range of motion and gradually add more weight in such exercises as squats, good mornings, and stiff-legged deadlifts. Increase the number of kicks in your workouts *gradually*.

Question: When one has a couple of days off—due to muscle soreness or just rest days—does it cause flexibility to decrease and set one back in training schedule?

Answer: Flexibility usually does not decrease much, and may even increase because of the rest the muscles got. If you do isometric stretches or any strength exercises even when you are sore because you are so anxious not to loose your flexibility temporarily, you may injure yourself and lose it permanently. You can do relaxed stretches, however, even if your muscles are sore as long as doing these stretches is not painful.

Question: I am 47 years old and I have had a total hip replacement for seven years (both my hip joints were damaged by Prednisone, which I had to take for Wegner Granulomatosis). I have been taking taekwondo lessons for more than two years. I cannot move either leg much past 90°, however. Please tell me how you feel I might progress in stretching with the video *Secrets of Stretching*.

Answer: I do not know if it is safe for you, with one hip replaced and the other damaged by Prednisone, to attempt the strenuous strength and flexibility exercises shown on *Secrets of Stretching.*

I recommend that you get yourself examined by an applied kinesiologist. My experience with them has been very good, and those that I have met are less conservative as far as exercise recommendations go and more knowledgeable, patient-oriented, and effective than all the orthopedic surgeons—"sports medicine specialists"— that ever treated me.

If you want to find an applied kinesiologist in your area, please call (913) 542-1801 or write to:

International College of Applied Kinesiology
P. O. Box 905
Lawrence, KS 66044

I sincerely hope that you will find a trustworthy doctor that will assist you in achieving your athletic goals.

Question: I purchased your book, and tape approximately one year ago and I have not achieved full splits yet. My hamstrings become extremely tight after attempting the splits but I have been experiencing less pain and soreness in the groin area on the next day. I have been using your isometric and relaxed stretches as part of my daily program with a break once or twice a week. I have avoided your dynamic stretches due to my back problem. I have been involved in karate for almost four years now (seven months ago I received my black belt in Shorin-Ryu karate at age 33). My diet includes a low fat vegetarian intake supplemented by ginseng, lecithin, selenium, royal bee jelly, spirulina, and vitamins C and E. I do have minor back and neck injuries, which are sources of intermittent pain and restriction.

Answer: Your inability to perform full splits after a full year of training may be caused by one of several factors.

a) Bad diet. Is your diet prescribed by a competent physician knowledgeable in sports medicine and sports nutrition? If not, consult with one! This diet may have something to do with your neck and back injuries and with hamstring tightness or weakness.

b) Your lower back problem may either affect the function of the muscles of your hips and thighs or prevent the proper positioning of the lower back and pelvis (forward tilt of the pelvis, see pages 15 and 17) that is necessary for performing a full split. Your hamstring tightness may also have a mechanical cause related to the lower back problem or be a result of lack of proper strength training.

c) You may be doing too much isometric stretching. You have stated that you stretch three times per day—I hope that does not mean that you perform isometric stretches in three sessions per day!

My advice to you is to seek the advice of an applied kinesiologist or of an osteopath and a nutritionist.

Question: I just recently pulled a hamstring in my right leg doing the front split. I rest it for a while till the pain is gone but it is the same thing all over again when I resume isometric stretches.

Answer: Apparently resting your injured hamstring does not remove the cause of the injury. Here is my advice concerning your hamstring.

a) See an applied kinesiologist, a chiropractor, or an orthopedic surgeon concerning your hamstring and do what your doctor advises you to do.

b) When permitted by your doctor, start doing the following exercises in this order: walking, climbing stairs, running uphill, squats, hamstring curls, stiff-legged deadlifts. Progress from one exercise to another only when feeling no discomfort performing the previous one.

c) Only after complete recovery (when hamstrings of both legs are equally strong, equally flexible, and have equal endurance) can you try isometric stretches involving hamstrings.

Question: I had a groin and hamstring pull that still bothers me. I would like to improve my flexibility, form, sparring ability, and balance in my spinning kicks. What are your suggestions?

Answer: Your objectives of improving flexibility, form, and sparring ability all depend on first treating *properly* your injuries. Before your hamstring and groin muscles are back in excellent working order no other work can be done. You need to see an applied kinesiologist or an *excellent* orthopedic surgeon (average to good may not suffice). After successful treatment, you may start working on strength and flexibility according to this book and the tape *Secrets of Stretching*. Develop balance in spinning kicks by performing spinning kicks at a low (below knee) target (initially imaginary, then soft, which will allow kicking/spinning through it). To strengthen your legs and prevent hamstring and groin injuries, do deadlifts and squats. Please consult weightlifting, powerlifting, or body-building manuals or see the video *Secrets of Stretching* for detailed description of these lifts.

Question: One day while stretching in a taekwondo dojang [gym] in Korea (I am in the Army), I was doing "butterflies" [see bottom picture on page 90]. When my instructor saw that my knees were not touching the floor, he came up behind me and forced them hard and quickly to the floor. The muscle was pulled in the left groin. Since then I have been very hesitant to stretch because of dull pain in that area. Maybe I'm doing something wrong?

Answer: Yes—you were doing something wrong. You were putting up with too much nonsense from a stupid "instructor." Now you should contact an applied kinesiologist and hope for the best.

Question: I am fifty-one years old, in good shape. For several years I have noticed that my right leg is much tighter than the left and recently I have noticed definite pain in the middle of the right buttock that also radiates down the leg. A week ago I was doing a static hamstring stretch sitting on the floor when I felt a stab of pain across my lower back. I have had pretty bad spasms ever since and I have trouble straightening up after sitting. Do you have any suggestions as to how can I overcome this and get back to training?

Answer: It looks like you have a lower back problem that was developing for several years—even before you first noticed that your right leg is tighter than the left. To find out when and if you can exercise again see an applied kinesiologist. The referral number of the International College of Kinesiology is on page 121.

Question: I have recently recovered from a low-back strain and have been told to do sit-ups, back extensions, and leg extensions to keep the muscles in this area strong. I would like to know if doing these exercises after my morning stretch would defeat the purpose of the dynamic and relaxed stretches?

Answer: No, these exercises would not ruin the effect of the stretches. To maximize the effect of both exercises and the stretches, you may start your morning with dynamic stretches, then do the exercises for your back, and then do relaxed stretches.

Question: On page 71 you state that people who experience knee problems should do strength exercises. What are these strength exercises?

Answer: Leg extensions, leg curls, squats, deadlifts.

Question: Although the book and the video go into depth about stretching, I found that they did not fully explain the stretches to be performed by those who suffer from "weak knees." What strength exercises will strengthen the muscles that stabilize the knee?

Answer: If your knees hurt when you do a stretch, change it so your knee bears less or no weight. For example, in hamstring or adductor stretches leading to a front or side split, place the lower end of your thigh on the chair or on any support. If bending your knees is not a problem you may do the exercises shown on page 71 and page 90.

The strength exercises that stabilize the knee are all those that affect muscles that originate above and attach below the knee joint. These exercises are squats, step-ups, deadlifts, good mornings, leg extensions, and leg flexions. If you cannot do these exercises because your knees were injured, then you can do isometric tensions with your knees held at angles at which you do not feel pain.

Question: I want to increase my vertical jump and maximize my flexibility. My coaches tell me I have to stretch my hamstrings, calf muscles and Achilles tendon to reach peak jumping ability. Is it true?

Answer: I do not think that improved flexibility of the legs will be of any help in jumping up.

If you want to know how to combine exercises developing strength, jumping ability, flexibility, and other abilities in your workouts for optimum results, please read *Science of Sports Training.*

Question: I would like to know how you feel about free weights for someone who plays tennis and is studying aikido. Do you recommend using free weights as a supplementary form of exercise for these athletic endeavors, or do you feel that doing all three forms of stretching is sufficient? If you do believe in using free weights, what routine would you recommend for the above sports?

Answer: Free weights are necessary in athletic training, even if the particular sport seems to require little strength, as a means of injury prevention and of preparing the body for intensive technical workouts. No stretches can replace free weights as a means of graduated resistance training. I cannot describe any "routine" for use of free weights in a letter because the choice of exercises depends on too many constantly changing factors for any routine to be useful and the lack of space and time prevents me from writing here about methodology of sports training. Instead, I recommend the video *Secrets of Stretching,* which covers the principles of general conditioning, strength, and flexibility training, or the book *Science of Sports Training.*

Question: I am a bodybuilder and I am using your stretching method. In your book on page 64 you show a weekly plan of workouts. Only one workout is dedicated to endurance. I thought that one should do aerobic exercises more often than that. Also, please tell me how I should combine your stretches with my bodybuilding exercises. I do my arms and chest on Monday and Friday, aerobics and then my legs on Tuesday and Saturday, my back on Wednesday, aerobics on Thursday, and I rest on Sunday.

Answer: Regarding aerobics—in the majority of sports and especially in contact sports such as boxing, judo, kickboxing, and wrestling, one main workout per week dedicated to purely aerobic endurance is usually enough because two (or more) technical workouts also stress all capabilities, aerobic capability among them, along with developing technical skills. Strength workouts also tend to have an endurance component—depending on the intensity of the workout or of particular exercises, the workout can be more anaerobic or more aerobic. Auxiliary workouts, short and done in addition to the main workout of the day, may be used to develop aerobic endurance.

Regarding your strength and flexibility training versus your bodybuilding routine—usually the legs (thighs) and the lower back are done in the same workout because of the necessary involvement of the lower back in all leg exercises. Because of its stabilizing function the lower back has to be done after all leg exercises.

Question: Are you aware of any long-term adverse effects of running or strength training on flexibility?

Answer: No, running or strength training have no adverse effect on flexibility provided you train rationally, do exercises in the correct sequence, and provide adequate rest to your body.

Question: Do you believe that larger muscles make you less flexible than smaller ones?

Answer: If you define flexibility as an ability to extend your joints maximally, then no—larger muscles do not make you less flexible. If you define flexibility as an ability to flex your joints, then yes—larger muscles can make you less flexible than smaller ones.

Question: Could you tell me what the cardiovascular warm-up is that you mention on page 30?

Answer: It is a part of the warm-up when you use continuous, low intensity, aerobic exercises to gradually prepare your heart and blood vessels for more intensive exercises.

Question: I do not know how to combine your flexibility exercises with my other physical activities. In a typical day in which I do everything, I would have the following timetable:
6:30 a.m.: rise and shine
7:30 a.m.: run 3-6 miles
9:00 a.m.: ride bicycle (30 min.) to work
6:00 p.m.: ride bicycle (30 min.) to hapkido class
7:00-9:00 p.m.: hapkido class (a Korean style of hand-to-hand combat with many kicks)
9:00 p.m.: ride bicycle (15 min.) home.
On weekends I do more cycling but this in one session. My flexibility is pitiful. Can you suggest a way of inserting the right type of stretches into my daily routine?

Answer: In your case doing all the stretches I recommend (dynamic in the morning, and at the beginning of your workout, static at the end of the workout) will not help if you keep riding your bike so much. Please see page 24 for the reason why cycling reduces flexibility. Also running 3-6 miles every morning may keep your legs tired and less responsive to stretching.

Question: I recently purchased your book and your video. I desire to follow your instructions to the letter (I refer to your advice against riding a bicycle for those that want great flexibility). My problem: Up to now I have been riding a bicycle for my cardiovascular workout! I live in a city apartment so jump rope and running without being on concrete are impractical. What is your suggestion?

Answer: Climb and eventually run up staircases.

Question: I want to know more about developing other physical abilities (strength, endurance, speed, coordination) and how they relate to flexibility. Would the book *Science of Sports Training* be helpful?

Answer: Yes.

Question: What is the difference between leg raises or front splits with the front leg straight and bent at the knee?

Answer: The angle between the thighs in a front split and in front raise (kick) is greater, or it is easier to increase it, when the front leg is bent at the knee because your hamstring is relaxed then. Exercise with your front leg straight to better stretch the hamstring.

Hamstrings originate *above* the hip joint and attach *below* the knee joint. Bending your knee relieves the tension of the hamstring and thus permits a greater range of movement in the hip joint. In a full front split, your pelvis is *always* tilted to the front *in relation* to the front thigh no matter what you do with your knees. Tilting of the pelvis is necessary for relaxing the ligamentum iliofemorale of the hip joint of the *rear thigh* (see page 15). You can achieve a greater amount of forward tilt when the knee of the front leg is bent because then the hamstring of your front leg is more relaxed.

Question: When you describe "leg raises," you refer to a slow, controlled lifting of the leg, not a quick swinging action, correct?

Answer: Controlled, yes, but not very slow.

Question: Is it better to take a shower before or after the morning stretch?

Answer: It should not matter. A few movements will warm you up better and faster than a hot shower, so you can save your time and shower only after the morning stretches.

Question: Can I do an early morning stretch after having my breakfast?

Answer: Yes, if you can perform a sufficient number of leg raises with adequate intensity and height without throwing up your breakfast.

Question: My bones pop and crack when I warm up and stretch. Is it dangerous?

Answer: Normally there is a bubble of air between joint surfaces so they do not rub each other. If the muscles crossing the joint are overly tensed this air bubble is squeezed out from between the joint surfaces and a vacuum forms in its place. The cracking sound is caused by air rushing in to fill this vacuum in a joint moved past its usual range of motion. Popping and cracking of joints is not harmful per se but *may* indicate some (perhaps excessive) tension of the muscles surrounding these joints. Another cause of sounds in a joint is osteoarthritis. When joint surfaces are diseased and the cartilage is eaten away, the ligaments and tendons crossing the joint get slack. Their slack lets them move in and out of their grooves, making popping sounds. See your chiropractor to make sure that all is okay.

Question: In chapter 3, "Dynamic Stretching," I am unsure how to perform the forward bends on page 49 and the bends to the back on page 50.

Answer: The answer to your question is in the chapter title itself. "*Dynamic* Stretching," right? Perform these movements in a controlled fashion but not very slow.

Question: Most of the stretches you show are practiced daily at my martial arts school. In fact most of them were taught to us in high school. Also, isometrics or dynamic tension is nothing new to this country. So why should your results be better?

Answer: It is not exercises alone that make the method effective. It is the way of arranging them in the proper sequence during a workout, during a day, and during a weekly cycle of workouts. Doing the same exercises in the wrong order reduces their effectiveness. I explain how various coordination, speed, strength, endurance, and flexibility exercises are influencing each other. Some exercises should follow each other and some should not.

Question: But sir, these stretches are the same we do at karate class five times a week, so why can't I do what you can?

Answer: It is not what exercises you do but, how, when, how much, and in what order. If you do isometric stretches five times a week then it is no wonder that you have difficulties with your flexibility, especially if you have to call on it without a warm-up.

Question: What is the difference between your book and your video on stretching? Do I need the video?

Answer: The book shows stretches for the whole body. It only mentions but does not show exercises other than stretches that develop strength and endurance while promoting flexibility. The book tells you all that you must know about flexibility but you have to devise your own exercise program on the basis of the provided (and abundant) information.

The video shows stretches as well as recommended endurance and strength exercises for your legs and trunk. The video is of the "do-along" type. If you do not know much about strength training, if your flexibility suffers because of lack of strength, if doing stretches makes your back tired, if you are often sore after a workout—then the video may help you.

Question: I have no access to an exercise machine to do adductor pull-downs (an adductor exercise shown in the video *Secrets of Stretching*). What can be done instead of this exercise?

Answer: You do not need an expensive exercise machine to do adductor pull-downs. You can attach a pulley to a beam or a tree and hang any type of weights at one end and make a loop for your foot at the other end. If that is impossible, you can do adductor flies with loads permitting about 10 repetitions.

Question: I practice karate and my teacher can lift a leg and hold it steady above his shoulder. Will your static active flexibility exercises let me achieve this type of strength so I can kick higher and with more power?

Answer: Yes and no. Static active flexibility exercises will help to develop your ability to lift and hold the leg but not to make your kicks more powerful. Specific strength for a kicker is the strength that lets one pack a wallop in a kick, not to hold a leg up! Specific strength for kicking is developed by kicking a heavy bag, kicking into layers of sponge, kicking with bungee cords attached to legs, and other dynamic exercises similar to kicking. Strength, just like flexibility, is specific to the speed of movement, its angle, and range of motion (McArdle, Katch and Katch 1991).

Question: When do I do dynamic stretches, when strength exercises, and when isometric stretches?

Answer: The answer to your question about dynamic stretches is on pages 30-31, 41-42; about strength workout and isometric stretches is on page 64.

But just in case you find the book difficult to follow, I will repeat it here. Do dynamic stretches at least twice per day, once in the morning and once during a warm-up for your workout.

Do strength training 2-3 times per week, ending with isometric stretches.

Question: I heard of a method of training called "dynamic tension." It involves performing various movements while simultaneously tensing all muscles. It is supposed to be very effective for developing strength and flexibility. What do you think of it?

Answer: It is difficult to gain as much strength with "dynamic tension" as with using external resistance, for example, weights, and this is why it is not used by weightlifters and track and field throwers. It is impossible to duplicate the character of effort and thus develop the specific strength and coordination required for any dynamic movement against resistance (wrestling, boxing, track and field) using "dynamic tension."

The way to evaluate "dynamic tension" is to compare the amount of time needed to achieve the same final results as with other methods, results such as the amount of strength in kicks and in static positions, or the ability to lift and hold a weight while sitting in a suspended split, for example.

To get the most out of your training I do not recommend you use any one method exclusively. Use all rational methods for the best overall result.

Question: Although I come within one foot of a full side split, my range of motion in dynamic stretches (when I swing my leg out to the side) is much worse. Why is this?

Answer: Make sure that you let your pelvis tilt forward (or move buttocks to the rear) when you raise your leg to the side. This action permits raising your leg higher—just as tilting your pelvis forward helps in the side split.

Question: Why does the body have a natural tendency to prevent one from doing a split? I know that I have the ability to do a split because when I do side lunges (one leg extended and one leg pulled in, supporting my body) I can do a "half-split." That is, I can fully extend one leg till my pelvis hits the floor—but with my other leg pulled in underneath me. I can do this with both legs but not at the same time. Why does the nervous system have to be trained to allow for fully extending both legs at the same time?

Answer: To find out more about the nervous system read about the reflexes in neurology textbooks or see page 22 in this book.

Apart from reflex contraction the lack of sufficient strength in adductors makes them tense harder and thus get shorter when both legs spread out have to support your weight. The wider the angle between your legs the less efficient is the adductors' leverage.

Question: Why don't you make a video for athletes who have a particular level of flexibility, for example, those who cannot reach their toes?

Answer: This method works regardless of anybody's level of flexibility. Exercises are demonstrated at a fairly high range of motion, but one can do them at any range, no matter how low, and increase it gradually.

Question: Would doing all stretches for all the body parts be too much flexibility training for karate?

Answer: I think it would be too much for any sport and for anybody's muscles.

Question: Is isometric stretching referred to as static stretching?

Answer: Isometric stretching is one of the varieties of static stretching.

Question: Could you suggest a program useful for karate?

Answer: I would suggest leg raises in all directions and isometric exercises for side and for front split.

Question: Would one or two months of not stretching reduce flexibility of someone who can do suspended splits?

Answer: I think that flexibility would not be reduced much but the strength in extended positions (suspended splits) would be too low to do them.

Question: Would doing weightlifting and all kinds of stretches in a workout be too much for one's muscles?

Answer: This depends on the person and exercises. If you do not feel sore after such workouts then they are probably okay.

Question: How long it takes to do full front and side splits using your book?

Answer: It depends on your strength and initial flexibility. Some people reach splits within a month while others need several months.

Question: I have found your book both inspiring and very helpful with my flexibility training. I weight train four times per week and I do gymnastics twice per week. My problem is that after I do leg exercises (leg presses, hack squats, but no regular squats due to the risk of injury) in my weight workout, my flexibility seems to go for about three to four days. Also my flexibility goes and then comes back again even without training. I do not know what causes it. I do not weight train excessively—one hour-and-a-half maximum per workout. I would like to achieve side and front splits and to be constantly flexible. Below I have written out my training schedule (obviously I am doing something wrong).

Sunday: Gymnastics (workout ends with relaxed stretches)

Monday: Weights (workout ends with static active flexibility exercises followed by isometric stretches)

Tuesday: Weights (workout ends with relaxed stretches)

Wednesday: Gymnastics (workout ends with relaxed stretches)

Thursday: Weights (workout ends with relaxed stretches)

Friday: Weights (workout ends with isometric stretches)

Saturday: Rest

Also my joints, especially hip and sacrum, are very "clicky" after workouts—is it dangerous?

Answer: You do not tell me how much you lift and on what days you do which lifts. You also do not tell me what exercises you do in your gymnastic workouts. Your problem may be caused by doing leg exercises too often, or not often enough. Here is a weekly schedule of workouts that you may want to try and see if it helps with your flexibility problems.

Sunday: Gymnastics (dynamic stretches in the warm-up; static active as needed; at the end of workout do isometric stretches for side splits with moderate tensions or, if legs too tired, do only relaxed stretches)

Monday: Weights (adductor exercises, leg presses, hack squats, good mornings, deadlifts, back extensions; do isometric stretches with strong tensions for side split either after adductor exercises or after hack squats but before lower back exercises)

Tuesday: Weights (arms, chest, upper back—use exercises that do not put compressive loads on your spine; end workout with relaxed stretches)

Wednesday: Gymnastics (dynamic stretches in the warm-up; static active as needed; at the end of workout do isometric stretches for side splits with moderate tensions or, if legs too tired, do only relaxed stretches)

Thursday: Weights (adductor exercises, leg presses, hack squats, good mornings, deadlifts, back extensions; do isometric stretches with strong tensions for side split either after adductor exercises or after hack squats but before lower back exercises)

Friday: Weights (arms, chest, upper back—use exercises that do not put compressive loads on your spine; end workout with relaxed stretches)

Saturday: Rest

See your doctor concerning the clicks in your joints.

Resources for Further Study

Science of Sports Training: How to Plan and Control Training for Peak Performance

by Thomas Kurz (Island Pond, VT: Stadion Publishing Company), 1991.

This comprehensive text delves deeply into topics such as speeding up recovery, using time- and energy-efficient training methods, avoiding overtraining and injuries, applying proven methods of training to specific sports, and maintaining a high level of condition and skills for years. The reader will learn ways to plan and control training for each workout, over a span of years.

Secrets of Stretching: Exercises for the Lower Body

(VHS videotape, 98 min.) featuring tom Kurz (Island Pond, VT: Stadion Publishing Company), 1990.

This video features an introduction to general conditioning and follows that with four exercise routines—one for beginners, one for intermediate, and two for advanced athletes. Viewers will learn plenty of how-tos. The focus is on flexibility and strength training.

Appendix: Normal Range of Joint Motion

Neck
Flexion 70-90° . . . . Touch sternum with chin.
Extension 55° . . . . Try to point up with chin.
Lateral bending 35° . . . . Bring ear close to shoulder.
Rotation 70° left & right. . . . . Turn head far to the left, then right.

Lumbar Spine
Flexion 75° . . . . Bend forward at the waist.
Extension 30° . . . . Bend backward.
Lateral bending 35° . . . . Bend to the side.

Shoulder
Abduction 180° . . . . Bring arm sideways up.
Adduction 45° . . . . Bring arm toward the midline of the body.
Horizontal extension 45° . . . . Swing arm horizontally backward.
Horizontal flexion 130° . . . . Swing arm horizontally forward.
Vertical extension 60° . . . . Raise arm straight backward.
Vertical flexion 180°. . . . . Raise arm straight forward.

Elbow
Extension 180° . . . . Straighten out lower arm.
Flexion 150° . . . . Bring lower arm to the biceps.
Supination 90° . . . . Turn lower arm so palm of the hand faces up.
Pronation 90° . . . . Turn lower arm so palm faces down.

Wrist
Flexion 80-90° . . . . Bend wrist so palm nears lower arm.
Extension 70° . . . . Bend wrist in opposite direction.
Radial deviation 20°. . . . . Bend wrist so thumb nears radius.
Ulnar deviation 30-50°. . . . . Bend wrist so small finger nears ulna.

Hip
Flexion 110-130° . . . . Flex knee and bring thigh close to abdomen.
Extension 30° . . . . Move thigh backward without moving pelvis.
Abduction 45-50°. . . . . Swing thigh away from midline.
Adduction 20-30°. . . . . Bring thigh toward and across the midline.
Internal rotation 40° . . . . Flex knee. Swing lower leg away from midline.
External rotation 45°. . . . . Flex knee. Swing lower leg toward midline.

Knee
Flexion 130° . . . . Touch calf to hamstring.
Extension 15° . . . . Straighten out knee as much as possible.
Internal rotation 10° . . . . Twist lower leg toward midline.

Ankle
Extension 20° . . . . Bend ankle so toes point up.
Flexion 45° . . . . Bend ankle so toes point down.
Pronation 30° . . . . Turn foot so the sole faces in.
Supination 20° . . . . Turn foot so the sole faces out.

Bibliography

Alter, M. J. 1988. *Science of Stretching*. Champaign: Human Kinetics Publishers, Inc.

Anderson, B. 1980. *Stretching*. Bolinas: Shelter Publications

Beighton, P., Grahame, R., Bird, H. 1983. *Hypermobility of joints*. Berlin: Springer-- Verlag

Bishop, B. 1982. *Basic Neurophysiology*. Garden City: Medical Examination Publishing Co.

Borowiec, S., Ronikier, A. 1977. *Zarys anatomii funkcjonalnej narzadow ruchu.* Warszawa: WAWF

Breit, N. J. 1977. *The effects of body position and stretching technique on development of hip and back flexibility*. Dissertation for degree of Doctor of Physical Education. Springfield College

Bullock, J., Boyle, J., Wang, M. B., Ajello R. R. 1984. *Physiology*. Media: Harval Publishing Co.

Burkett, L. N. 1968. *Causative factors in hamstring strains*. Master of Arts thesis. San Diego State College

Chrominski, Z. 1980. *Metodyka sportu dzieci i mlodziezy*. Warszawa: Sport i Turystyka

deVries, H. A. 1980. *Physiology of Exercise for Physical Education and Athletics*. Dubuque: Wm. C. Brown Company Publishers

Etnyre, B. R., Abraham, L. D. 1986. "Reflex changes during static stretching and two variations of proprioceptive neuromuscular facilitation techniques" *Electroencephalography and Clinical Neurophysiology* 63:174-178

Fox, E. L. 1979. *Sports Physiology*. Philadelphia: Saunders College Publishing

Fridén, J. 1984. "Changes in human skeletal muscle induced by long-term eccentric exercise." *Cell and Tissue Research* 236(2):365-372

Giesielievich, B. A. 1976. *Medicinskii spravochnik trieniera*. Moskva: Fizkultura i Sport

Grochmal, S. 1979. *Teoria i metodyka cwiczen relaksowo- koncentrujacych*. Warszawa: PZWL

Hettinger, T., Müller, E. A. 1953 "Muskelleistung und Muskeltraining." *Arbeitsphysiologie* 15:111-126

Hill, A. V. 1961. "The heat produced by a muscle after the last shock of tetanus." *Journal of Physiology* 159:518-545

Johns, R. J., Wright, V. 1962. "Relative importance of various tissues in joint stiffness." *Journal of Applied Physiology* 17:824-28

Knots, M., Voss, D. E. 1968. *PNF Patterns and Techniques*. New York: Harper and Row

Knuttgen, H. G. 1976. *Neuromuscular Mechanisms for Therapeutic and Conditioning Exercise*. Baltimore: University Park Press

Kukushkin, G. I. 1983. *Sistiema fizichieskovo vospitania v SSSR*. Moskva: Raduga

Leighton, J. R. 1964. "A study of the effect of progressive weight training on flexibility." *American Corrective Therapy Journal* 18(4):101

Licht, S. 1965. *Therapeutic Exercise*. Baltimore: Waverley Press, Inc.

MacConail, M. A., Basmajian, J. V. 1969. *Muscles and Movements, A Basis for Human Physiology*. Baltimore: The Williams and Wilkins Co.

Matvyeyev, L. P. 1977. *Osnovy sportivnoy trienirovki*. Moskva: Fizkultura i Sport

McArdle, W. D., Katch, F. I., Katch, V. L. 1991. *Exercise Physiology: Energy, Nutrition, and Human Performance.* Malvern: Lea & Febiger

Moore, M. A., Kukulka, C. G. 1991. "Depression of Hoffman reflexes following voluntary contraction and implications for proprioceptive neuromuscular facilitation therapy." *Physical Therapy* 71(4):321-329

Müller, E. A., Röhmert, W. 1963 "Die Geschwindigkeit der Muskelkraft—Zunahme bei isometrischen Training." *Arbeitsphysiologie* 19:403-419

Naglak, Z. 1979. *Trening sportowy—Teoria i praktyka.* Warszawa: PWN

Potter, P. A. 1985. *Pocket Nurse Guide to Physical Assessment.* St.Louis: The C. V. Mosby Company

Ramsey, R. W., Street, S. F. 1940. "Isometric length tension diagram of isolated skeletal muscle fibers of the frog." *Journal of Cellular and Comparative Physiology* 15:11

Roberts, T. D. M. 1978. *Neurophysiology of postural mechanisms.* Boston: The Butterworth Group

Russe, O. A., Gerhardt, J. J., King, T. C. 1972. *An Atlas of Examination, Standard Measurements and Diagnosis in Orthopedics and Traumatology.* Baltimore: The Williams and Wilkins Co.

Schottelius, B. A., Senay, L. C. 1956. "Effect of stimulation-length sequence on shape of length-tension diagram." *American Journal of Physiology* 186:127-130

Sölveborn, S. A. 1989. *Stretching.* Warszawa: Sport i Turystyka

Ulatowski, T. 1979. *Teoria i metodyka sportu.* Warszawa: WAWF

Wallis, E. L., Logan, G. A. 1964. *Figure improvement and body conditioning through exercise.* Englewood Cliffs: Prentice-Hall

Wickstrom, R. L. 1963. "Weight training and flexibility." *Journal of Health, Physical Education and Recreation* 34(2):61-62

Wolf, J. K. 1980. *Practical Clinical Neurology.* Garden City: Medical Examination Publishing Co.

Index